MCQs 3-in-1
BASIC HEALTH NURSING

MCQs 3-in-1
BASIC HEALTH NURSING

Second Edition

Rajeswari Vaidyanathan
MSc (N) PhD
Former Principal
Madras Medical College
Chennai, Tamil Nadu, India

Foreword
R Indira

JAYPEE The Health Sciences Publisher
New Delhi | London | Panama

Jaypee Brothers Medical Publishers (P) Ltd

Headquarters

Jaypee Brothers Medical Publishers (P) Ltd.
4838/24, Ansari Road, Daryaganj
New Delhi 110 002, India
Phone: +91-11-43574357
Fax: +91-11-43574314
Email: jaypee@jaypeebrothers.com

Overseas Offices

J.P. Medical Ltd.
83, Victoria Street, London
SW1H 0HW (UK)
Phone: +44-20 3170 8910
Fax: +44-(0)20 3008 6180
Email: info@jpmedpub.com

Jaypee-Highlights Medical Publishers Inc.
City of Knowledge, Bld. 235, 2nd Floor, Clayton
Panama City, Panama
Phone: +1 507-301-0496
Fax: +1 507-301-0499
Email: cservice@jphmedical.com

Jaypee Brothers Medical Publishers (P) Ltd.
Bhotahity, Kathmandu, Nepal
Phone: +977-9741283608
Email: kathmandu@jaypeebrothers.com

Jaypee Brothers Medical Publishers (P) Ltd.
17/1-B, Babar Road, Block-B, Shaymali
Mohammadpur, Dhaka-1207
Bangladesh
Mobile: +08801912003485
Email: jaypeedhaka@gmail.com

Website: www.jaypeebrothers.com
Website: www.jaypeedigital.com

Inquiries for bulk sales may be solicited at: jaypee@jaypeebrothers.com

MCQs 3-in-1 Basic Health Nursing

First Edition: **2006**

Second Edition: **2017**

ISBN: **978-93-86322-15-9**

Printed at

Dedicated to

Mr V Vaidyanathan
Mr Girivas Vaidyanathan and
Mrs Mahalakshmi Girivas
Mr Magesh Vaidyanathnan and Dr Arthi Magesh

Grandchildren

Master Hari Girivas and Sri Ram Girivas
Ms Isha Magesh and Master Arjun Magesh
and
My dear everloving nursing students.

Foreword

'Nursing' as a profession has to move to new heights in the delivery of nursing services at par with the advancing scientific technology era. To this, nursing education has to progress to provide scientific knowledge to render standard care in clinical practice.

Prof Dr Rajeswari Vaidyanathan, being a clinical nurse educator, administrator and researcher has been associated with nursing at various levels in Chennai, Tamil Nadu, India, for more than four decades.

I am very proud to say that I did my PG program under her. This book is written in a simpler manner for the nursing students, who are undergoing for GNM and BSc Nursing programs.

I hope this book will increase knowledge of nursing students and which will also be beneficial for their bright future.

Prof R Indira
Dean
Narayana Nursing Institute
Nellore, Andhra Pradesh, India

Preface to the Second Edition

For BSc(N) university examination, some universities had introduced the Multiple Choice Questions as one section in some states.

The students of nursing face difficulty in finding complete and comprehensive answers in books. For the convenience of the students, this second edition of *MCQs 3-in-1 Basic Health Nursing* will be a guide to fulfill their requirements to face the examination successfully.

This book will be of great benefit to the nursing students of I, II and IV years appearing for the subjects, Nursing Foundation, Community Health Nursing and Nursing Education to get through the University Examination scoring highest marks in all the above subjects.

Rajeswari Vaidyanathan

Preface to the First Edition

Dr MGR Medical University has recently introduced the trend of Multiple Choice Questions in the examination pattern.

The students of Nursing face great difficulty in finding a complete and comprehensive answers in voluminous books. For the convenience of the students as well as to fulfill the requirement of the examination pattern, I have written this MCQs book.

It is hoped that this book will be of great benefit to the Nursing students, which would make students understand about the subject quite clear.

Rajeswari Vaidyanathan

Acknowledgments

In my professional life, I have climbed the career-ladder starting with Clinical Nurse, Nurse Educator and Nurse Administrator in both Nursing Colleges and Directorate of Medical Education. I had taken opportunities to teach all the above subjects to the nursing students and understood their difficulties to face the MCQs section which in turn motivated me to bring this book to dedicate my everloving nursing students.

I am grateful to Sh Jitendar P Vij (Group Chairman) of M/s Jaypee Brothers Medical Publishers (P) Ltd., the Editorial Board and the publishing division, who have given their full support to bring out this essential nursing book. Mr R Jayanandan (Author Co-ordinator), Chennai Branch, always encouraged me as a backbone and his timely help motivated me to bring out this book.

Contents

CHAPTER 1

Nursing Foundation

1. **Health is:**
   A. The absence of illness
   B. The opposite of disease
   C. A condition between disease and good health
   D. A state of complete physical, mental and social well-being

2. **A person's state of health, wellness or illness depends on an individuals:**
   A. Self concept
   B. Lifestyle
   C. Known risk factors
   D. Values and personality

3. **The relationship between health and illness in the health-illness continuum model is:**
   A. Stable
   B. Stagnant
   C. Dynamic
   D. Developing

4. **Health belief in health-belief model usually influence:**
   A. Health status
   B. Health outcomes
   C. Health behaviours
   D. Health determinants

5. **The health-promotion model attempts to explain the:**
   A. Effect of environment on an individual
   B. Effect of health activity on an individual
   C. Reasons individuals avoid health activities
   D. Reasons individuals engage in health activities

---

1 D 2 A 3 B 4 C 5 D

6. **Holistic health interventions are used to:**
   A. Replace standard medical therapy
   B. Improve standard medical therapy
   C. Compliment standard medical therapy
   D. Compete with standard medical therapy

7. **The health status of an individual or community is:**
   A. Multifactorial
   B. One dimensional
   C. Determined by genetics
   D. Determined by environment

8. **Health promotion activities are activities that:**
   A. Treat disease
   B. Prevent illness
   C. Help maintain or enhance health
   D. Protect against health threats

9. **Primary prevention strategy is:**
   A. Identify disease problems
   B. Treat chronic diseases
   C. Reduces the severity of illness
   D. Disease vulnerability to illness

10. **The presence of certain risk factors:**
    A. Have no roll in health practices
    B. Suggest that a disease will definitely develop
    C. Increase the chance the disease will develop
    D. Decrease the chance the disease will progress

11. **An illness in a family member affects the function of the:**
    A. Siblings
    B. Parent diet
    C. Individual only
    D. Entire family unit

12. **Pre-natal care/well baby care/nutrition counseling/family planning/exercise classes are example for:**
    A. Primary care
    B. Secondary care
    C. Tertiary care
    D. Restorative care

---

6 C 7 A 8 C 9 D 10 C 11 A 12 A

13. **Blood pressure and cancer screening/immunizations/crisis prevention/mental health counseling are example for:**
    A. Primary care
    B. Secondary care
    C. Tertiary care
    D. Restorative care

14. **Cardiovascular and pulmonary rehabilitation/spinal cord injury programmes/sports medicine/home health care are example for:**
    A. Primary care
    B. Secondary care
    C. Continuing care
    D. Restorative care

15. **The most common source of injury to patient is:**
    A. Pressure sore
    B. Burns from heart liquids
    C. Offering chipped bed pan
    D. Falls

16. **Obtaining informed consent is the responsibility of the:**
    A. Patient
    B. Physician
    C. Student nurse
    D. Head nurse

17. **The legal definition of death that facilitates organ donation is:**
    A. Cessation of pulse
    B. Cessation of respirations
    C. Cessation of circulatory and respiratory functions
    D. Cessation of function of the entire brain

18. **The code of ethics for nurses is composed and published by the:**
    A. National League for Nursing
    B. American Nurses Association
    C. American Medical association
    D. National Institution of Health

---

13 B   14 D   15 D   16 B   17 D   18 B

19. **Autonomy refers to:**
    A. Person's independence
    B. Responsibility
    C. Accountability
    D. Fidelity

20. **Principle of fairness is:**
    A. Autonomy
    B. Fidelity
    C. Justice
    D. Advocacy

21. **The agreement to keep promises is the:**
    A. Autonomy
    B. Fidelity
    C. Justice
    D. Advocacy

22. **Taking positive active steps to help others is the:**
    A. Beneficence
    B. Non-maleficence
    C. Responsibility
    D. Accountability

23. **Non-maleficence refers to the:**
    A. Fundamental agreement to do no harm
    B. Taking positive active steps to help others
    C. Agreement to keep promises
    D. Persons independence

24. **The execution of duties associated with a nurse's particular role is the:**
    A. Autonomy
    B. Fidelity
    C. Accountability
    D. Responsibility

25. **Ability to answer for nurse's actions is the:**
    A. Autonomy
    B. Accountability
    C. Responsibility
    D. Respectivity

---

19 A 20 C 21 B 22 A 23 A 24 C 25 B

26. **The identification of client's health care needs occurs in the nursing process step of:**
    A. Planning
    B. Evaluation
    C. Assessment
    D. Implementation

27. **The most important skills needed to obtain accurate information by a nurse from a patient are:**
    A. Teaching skills
    B. Cognitive skills
    C. Psychomotor skills
    D. Interpersonal skills

28. **Before formulating a list of nursing diagnosis, a nurse must first:**
    A. Establish a list of priorities
    B. Document assessment of findings
    C. Review assessment with health team members
    D. Validate physical examination findings

29. **Establishing priorities for patients had occurs in the nursing process step are:**
    A. Planning
    B. Evaluation
    C. Assessment
    D. Implementation

30. **Nursing diagnosis is formulated by:**
    A. SNA B. ANA
    C. TNA D. INC

31. **Nursing diagnosis is formulated once in:**
    A. 2 years B. 3 years
    C. 4 years D. 5 years

32. **The most crucial stage of the nursing process is:**
    A. Assessment
    B. Planning
    C. Intervention
    D. Evaluation

---

26 C 27 D 28 D 29 A 30 B 31 A 32 A

33. **Taking nursing history comes in:**
    A. Assessment B. Planning
    C. Intervention D. Evaluation

34. **Providing nursing care or actual nursing care comes in:**
    A. Assessment B. Planning
    C. Intervention D. Evaluation

35. **Measuring outcomes of nursing care comes in:**
    A. Assessment B. Planning
    C. Intervention D. Evaluation

36. **Feeling of internal organs by hands is the:**
    A. Palpation
    B. Auscultation
    C. Inspection
    D. Manipulation

37. **The intended goal of incident reports is to:**
    A. Provide information in the medical record
    B. Reprimand individuals in the incident
    C. Identify changes needed to prevent reoccurrence
    D. Document actual injury and follow-up action

38. **The information that objective data:**
    A. Information about education
    B. A description of joint mobility
    C. Assessment of breath sounds
    D. A description of pain

39. **Active listening is demonstrated by:**
    A. Agreeing with the client
    B. Repeating everything the client says to clarify
    C. Assuming a relaxed posture and leaning toward the client
    D. Smiling and nodding throughout the interview

40. **Ethical dilemmas can best be solved by:**
    A. Relationship
    B. Ethical principles
    C. Homecare nurses
    D. Code of ethics for nurses

---

33 A 34 C 35 D 36 A 37 C 38 C 39 C
40 A

41. When nursing an older adult, nurse should remember to avoid:

A. Touching the client
B. Shifting from subject to subject
C. Allowing the client to remain quite
D. Asking the client how he or she feels

42. When rendering nursing care to a client who is unresponsive, a nurse should remember to:

A. Speak lovely
B. Use touch sparingly
C. Used the client's name and explain procedures
D. Spent as little time as possible

43. The most effective way to break the chain of infection is by:

A. Hand washing
B. Wearing clouse
C. Placing patient in isolation
D. Providing private rooms for all patients

44. Indwelling urinary catheter represents a risk for urinary tract infection because it:

A. Keep an incontinent patient's skin dry
B. Can get cot in the linens
C. Obstructs the normal fleshing action of urine flow
D. Allows the patient to remain hydrated

45. Gloves should be removed and hands washed:

A. Only after home care
B. When leaving the room
C. After completing all care for the patient
D. When the specific task is completed

46. Vital signs of respiration 8 and heart rate 46/minute is described as:

A. Bradycardia and apnea
B. Tachycardia and apnea
C. Bradycardia and bradypnea
D. Tachycardia and bradypnea

41 A 42 C 43 A 44 C 45 D 46 C

47. **A pulse deficit is:**
    A. The difference between the radial and apical pulse rate
    B. The digital pressure felt when taking radial pulse
    C. The amount of pressure felt when taking radial pulse
    D. The amount of pressure felt when taking ulnar pulse

48. **In too narrow or too loose wrapped BP cuff, BP will be:**
    A. Falsely low
    B. Falsely high
    C. Hear muffled sounds
    D. Depends on the examiner's hearing acquity

49. **Application of cool clothes to the auxilla, to decrease the body temperature through:**
    A. Conduction
    B. Convection
    C. Evaporation
    D. Radiation

50. **Removing excess blankets from the patient to decrease the body temperature through:**
    A. Conduction
    B. Convection
    C. Evaporation
    D. Radiation

51. **Fever spikes and falls without a return to normal is:**
    A. Sustained fever
    B. Remittent fever
    C. Intermittent fever
    D. Relapsing fever

52. **The most important sign of heat stroke is:**
    A. Hot dry skin
    B. Cold dry skin
    C. Hot moist skin
    D. Cold moist skin

53. **Oxygen saturation is measured by:**
    A. Pulse oximeter
    B. Thermometer
    C. Manometer
    D. Pulse transducer

54. **Poor oxygenation of the blood will affect and cause the pulse to become:**
    A. Bounding
    B. Irregular
    C. Faster
    D. Slower

---

47 A 48 B 49 A 50 D 51 B 52 A 53 A
54 C

55. **Increased pulse rate than normal is:**
A. Tachycardia B. Bradycardia
C. Tachypnea D. Bradypnea

56. **Decreased pulse rate than normal is:**
A. Tachycardia B. Bradycardia
C. Tachypnea D. Bradypnea

57. **Increased respiratory rate than normal is:**
A. Tachycardia B. Bradycardia
C. Tachypnea D. Bradypnea

58. **Decreased respiratory rate than normal is:**
A. Tachycardia B. Bradycardia
C. Tachypnea D. Bradypnea

59. **Difference between the systolic and diastolic pressure is:**
A. Pulse pressure B. Pulse deficit
C. Cardiac output D. Blood pressure

60. **Cardinal symptom includes:**
A. Temperature pulse and respiration
B. Temperature and pulse
C. Temperature and respiration
D. Pulse and respiration

61. **Water hammer pulse is also known as:**
A. Corrigan's pulse
B. Collapsing pulse
C. Running pulse
D. Bounding pulse

62. **A jerky pulse with full expansion followed by sudden collapse is:**
A. Collapsing pulse
B. Corrigan's pulse
C. Running pulse
D. Bounding pulse

63. **Difficulty to breathe in lying down is:**
A. Orthopnea B. Dyspnea
C. Apnea D. Bradypnea

---

55 A 56 B 57 C 58 D 59 A 60 A 61 A
62 B 63 A

64. **Cessation of breathing for a short period is:**
    A. Orthopnea
    B. Dyspnea
    C. Apnea
    D. Bradypnea

65. **The first technique to be employed when performing a client's physical examination is:**
    A. Palpation
    B. Inspection
    C. Percussion
    D. Auscultation

66. **To assess the patient's posterior tibial pulse, a nurse would palpate:**
    A. Behind the knee
    B. Over the medial malleolus
    C. Below the medial malleolus
    D. Below the lateral malleolus

67. **To assess the patient's popliteal pulse, a nurse would palpate:**
    A. Behind the knee
    B. Over the knee
    C. Above the knee
    D. Below the knee

68. **The main reason of auscultating abdomen before palpation in physical examination is to:**
    A. Prevent distortion of vascular sounds
    B. Prevent distortion of bowel sounds
    C. Determined any areas of tenderness
    D. Allow the patient to relax

69. **To correctly palpate the patient's skin for temperature, a nurse will use the:**
    A. Base of hands
    B. Fingertips of hands
    C. Dorsal surface of hands
    D. Palmar surface of hands

70. **To assess a client's superficial lymph nodes, a nurse would:**
    A. Deeply palpate using entire hand
    B. Deeply palpate using a bi-manual technique
    C. Likely using a bi-manual technique
    D. Gently using the birds of index and middle fingers

64 C 65 B 66 C 67 A 68 B 69 C 70 D

71. **To spread the breast tissue evenly over the chest wall during an examination, a nurse ask the patient to lie supine with:**
 A. Hands clasped just above the abdomen
 B. Both arms overhead
 C. Both arms along the body
 D. One arm behind the head

72. **To palpate the upper outer quadrant of breast tissue is important because this area is:**
 A. The largest area of the breast
 B. More prone to calcification
 C. Where most breast tumours are located
 D. Where most lymph nodes are located

73. **A nurse teach the patient to inspect all skin surfaces and to report pigmented skin lesions that:**
 A. Are symmetrical
 B. Have irregular borders
 C. Are uniform in colour
 D. Are less than 6 mm in diameter

74. **For assessing range of joint movement, a nurse ask the patient to move the arm away from the body evaluating the movement of:**
 A. Flexion
 B. Extension
 C. Abduction
 D. Adduction

75. **When inspecting the patient's anterior thorax, a nurse observe for:**
 A. Presence of fremitus
 B. Presence of breath sounds
 C. Movement of the diaphragm
 D. Symmetry of chest excursion

76. **When auscultating the adult patient's thorax, a nurse would:**
 A. Instruct him to take deep rapid breaths
 B. Instruct him to breathe in and out through the nose
 C. Use the bell of the stethoscope
 D. Use the diaphragm of the stethoscope

71 D 72 A 73 B 74 C 75 C 76 B

77. **The systematic pattern to be used for comparison when auscultating the patients lung fields is:**
    A. Side to side
    B. Top to bottom
    C. Anterior to posterior
    D. Interface to interface

78. **When testing sensory pathways, a nurse:**
    A. Use a predictable order
    B. Perform each test quickly
    C. Compare symmetrical areas
    D. Allow the patient's eyes remain open

79. **Asking the patient to smile, frown and raise and lower the eyebrows to test the action of the cranial nerves is:**
    A. Facial
    B. Trigeminal
    C. Oculomotor
    D. Hypoglossar

80. **A 3+ reflex grade in reflex test indicates the:**
    A. Normal
    B. Hyperactive
    C. Below normal
    D. Brisker than normal

81. **To examine for hernias a nurse ask the patient to:**
    A. Jump in place
    B. Lift a heavy object
    C. Strain or beardown
    D. Assume the prone positions

82. **Hearing of S_1 sound best at the apex core relates with closure of the:**
    A. Aortic and mitral valves
    B. Mitral and tricuspid valves
    C. Aortic and pulmonary valves
    D. Tricuspid and pulmonary valves

83. **When conducting an otoscopic examination on an infant, a nurse:**
    A. Release the auricle once the speculum is in place
    B. Use the largest speculum
    C. Pull the auricle up and back before inserting the speculum
    D. Pull the auricle down and back before inserting the speculum

---

77 A 78 C 79 A 80 D 81 D 82 A 83 D

84. **The position used to assess the extension of hip joint is:**
A. Supine B. Prone
C. Sitting D. Dorsal recumbent

85. **The position that provides maximal exposure of rectal area is:**
A. Supine B. Prone
C. Knee chest D. Lithotomy

86. **The position provides maximal exposure of genetalia and facilitates insertion of veginal speculum is:**
A. Dorsal recumbent B. Lithotomy
C. Simps D. Knee chest

87. **The position provides easy access to pulse sites is:**
A. Prone B. Supine
C. Sitting D. Dorsal recumbent

88. **The position used for abdominal assessment is:**
A. Prone B. Supine
C. Dorsal recumbent D. Lateral recumbent

89. **Flat nonpalpable change in skin colour smaller than 1 cm skin lesion is the:**
A. Macule B. Papule
C. Vesicle D. Nodule

90. **Palpable solid elevation in skin smaller than 0.5 cm skin lesion is the:**
A. Macule B. Papule
C. Vesicle D. Nodule

91. **Elevated solid mass deeper and firmer than papule 0.2 to 0.5 cm skin lesion is the:**
A. Macule
B. Vesicle
C. Nodule
D. Pustule

92. **The normal angle between nail plate and nail is:**
A. 160 B. 140
C. 180 D. 120

---

84 B 85 C 86 B 87 B 88 C 89 A 90 B
91 C 92 A

93. The angle between nail plate and nail more than 180 seen in:
A. Normal nail
B. Clubbing
C. Paronychia
D. Koilonychia

94. Inflammation of skin at base of nail is:
A. Clubbing
B. Paronychia
C. Koilonychia
D. Bean's limes

95. Dropping of the eyelid is called:
A. Ptosis
B. Otitis
C. Ectropion
D. Entropion

96. Turn out of the lid margins is called:
A. Ptosis
B. Otitis
C. Ectropion
D. Entropion

97. Turn in of the lid margins is known as:
A. Ptosis
B. Otitis
C. Ectropion
D. Entropion

98. If assessment of pupilary reaction is normal in all test, the abbreviation used to record is:
A. PERRLA
B. SEARLA
C. SEROSA
D. PERLA

99. Vibrations created by the sound waves that is created by the vocal cords transmitted through the lung to the chest wall are called:
A. Tactile fremitis
B. Crackles
C. Adventitious sounds
D. Sibilent wheeze

100. Prolonged intake of medication or accumulation of medication in the blood causes:
A. Side effect
B. Adverse effect
C. Toxic effect
D. Therapeutic effect

93 B 94 B 95 A 96 C 97 D 98 D 99 A
100 C

101. Preparation usually containing alcohol, oil or soapy emollient, i.e. applied to skin is:
A. Liniment B. Lotion
C. Oilment D. Solution

102. Drug in liquid suspension applied to protect skin is:
A. Liniment B. Lotion
C. Oilment D. Solution

103. Predictable, unintended secondary effects caused by a medication is the:
A. Side effect
B. Adverse effect
C. Toxic effect
D. Therapeutic effect

104. One medication modifies the action of another medication is the:
A. Medication interaction
B. Allergic reaction
C. Idiosyncratic reaction
D. Medication allergic

105. Unpredictable effects in which a patient over-acts or under reacts to a medication is the:
A. Idiosyncratic reaction
B. Allergic reaction
C. Anaphylactic reaction
D. Medication interaction

106. Severe responses to medication is the:
A. Side effect
B. Adverse effect
C. Toxic effect
D. Therapeutic effect

107. In medication administration, stat means:
A. Give immediately
B. Give before meals
C. Give as desired
D. Give after meals

---

101 A 102 B 103 A 104 A 105 A 106 B 107 A

108. **In medication administration, prn means:**
   A. Give when needed
   B. Give before meals
   C. Give after meals
   D. Give immediately

109. **The abbreviation used when medication to be given before meals is:**
   A. ac
   B. ad lib
   C. pc
   D. hs

110. **The abbreviation used when medication to be given as desired is:**
   A. ac
   B. ad lib
   C. pc
   D. hs

111. **The abbreviation hs denotes the administration of medication is:**
   A. Before meals
   B. After meals
   C. At night
   D. As needed

112. **A medication given under the tongue is:**
   A. Sublingual
   B. Subcutaneous
   C. Transdermal
   D. Buccal

113. **In buccal administration, the solid medication to be placed against the:**
   A. Mouth and mucous membrane
   B. Tongue and mucous membrane
   C. Tongue
   D. Mouth

114. **Suppository to be administered into the:**
   A. Mouth
   B. Nose
   C. Rectum
   D. Ear

115. **A patient is to receive cephalixin— 500 mg po. The pharmacy has sent 250 mg tablets. The nurse should give:**
   A. Half tablet
   B. One tablet
   C. 1½ tablet
   D. 2 tablets

---

108 A 109 A 110 B 111 C 112 A 113 B 114 C
115 D

116. The patient has an order for 2 table spoon of milk of magnesia. The nurse would give:
A. 2 ml B. 5 ml
C. 16 ml D. 20 ml

117. Positively charged electrolytes are:
A. Solvent B. Solution
C. Cations D. Anions

118. An element or compound able to carry an electric current is:
A. Electrolyte B. Mixture
C. Acid D. Alkali

119. A process in which a solute in a solution moves from an area of higher concentration to an area of lower concentration is:
A. Diffusion B. Osmosis
C. Infiltration D. Ultrafiltration

120. A solution of higher osmotic pressure that pull fluid from cells is:
A. Isotonic B. Hypotonic
C. Hypertonic D. Oncotic

121. A solution expand a body's fluid volume without causing a fluid shift from one compartment to another is:
A. Isotonic B. Hypotonic
C. Hypertonic D. Oncotic

122. A solution of lower oncotic pressure that moves into the cells causing them to enlarge is:
A. Isotonic B. Hypotonic
C. Hypertonic D. Oncotic

123. An excessive vomiting and haemorrhage leads to:
A. Hypovolaemia B. Hypervolaemia
C. Fluid overload D. Oedema

124. A substance or group of substances that can absorb or release H^+ to correct an acid base imbalance is:
A. Buffer B. Anion
C. Cation D. Renin

116 D 117 C 118 A 119 A 120 C 121 A 122 B
123 A 124 A

125. **Increased sweating leads to:**
A. Hyponatremia
B. Hypernatremia
C. Hypervolaemia
D. Oedema

126. **Increased sensible and insensible water loss leads to:**
A. Hyponatremia
B. Hypernatremia
C. Hypervolaemia
D. Oedema

127. **Fluid volume deficit causes:**
A. Hypokalaemia
B. Hyperkalaemia
C. Hypocalcaemia
D. Hypercalcaemia

128. **Diarrhea, vomitting and other gastric fluid losses cause:**
A. Hypokalaemia
B. Hyperkalaemia
C. Hypocalcaemia
D. Hypercalcaemia

129. **Rapid administration of blood transfusions containing citrate causes:**
A. Hypokalaemia
B. Hyperkalaemia
C. Hypocalcaemia
D. Hypercalcaemia

130. **Prolonged immobilization causes:**
A. Hypokalaemia
B. Hyperkalaemia
C. Hypocalcaemia
D. Hypercalcaemia

131. **Excess oral or parenteral intake of magnesium causes:**
A. Hypocalcaemia
B. Hypercalcaemia
C. Hypomagnesemia
D. Hypermagnesemia

132. **Heavy loss of acid from the body or by increased levels of bi-corbonate causes:**
A. Metabolic acidosis
B. Metabolic alkalosis
C. Respiratory acidosis
D. Respiratory alkalosis

133. **High acid content of the blood results in:**
A. Metabolic acidosis
B. Metabolic alkalosis
C. Respiratory acidosis
D. Respiratory alkalosis

---

125 A 126 B 127 B 128 A 129 C 130 D 131 D
132 B 133 A

134. Hypoventilation leads to:
- A. Metabolic acidosis
- B. Metabolic alkalosis
- C. Respiratory acidosis
- D. Respiratory alkalosis

135. Hyperventilation leads to:
- A. Metabolic acidosis
- B. Metabolic alkalosis
- C. Respiratory acidosis
- D. Respiratory alkalosis

136. Dextrose 5% in water is an example for:
- A. Isotonic solution
- B. Hypotonic solution
- C. Hypertonic solution
- D. None of these

137. Dextrose 10% in water is an example for:
- A. Isotonic solution
- B. Hypotonic solution
- C. Hypertonic solution
- D. None of these

138. Lactated Ringers solution is an example for:
- A. Isotonic solution
- B. Hypotonic solution
- C. Hypertonic solution
- D. None of these

139. Dextrose 5% in Lactated Ringer solution is an example for:
- A. Isotonic solution
- B. Hypotonic solution
- C. Hypertonic solution
- D. None of these

140. 0.45% sodium chloride solution is an example for:
- A. Isotonic solution
- B. Hypotonic solution
- C. Hypertonic solution
- D. None of these

---

134 C 135 D 136 A 137 C 138 A 139 C 140 B

141. 0.09% sodium chloride solution in an example for:

A. Isotonic solution
B. Hypotonic solution
C. Hypertonic solution
D. None of these

142. Dextrose 5% in 0.45% sodium chloride solution is an example for:

A. Isotonic solution
B. Hypotonic solution
C. Hypertonic solution
D. None of these

143. Dextrose 5% in 0.9% sodium chloride is an example for:

A. Isotonic solution
B. Hypotonic solution
C. Hypertonic solution
D. None of these

144. 3 or 5% sodium chloride is an example for:

A. Isotonic solution
B. Hypotonic solution
C. Hypertonic solution
D. None of these

145. The patient at greatest risk for fluid volume excess is a:

A. 20-year-old patient with 3 years history of diabetes mellitus
B. 86-year-old patient with fractured pelvis
C. 49-year-old patient with second degree burns
D. 60-year-old patient with congestive heart failure

146. When providing for a patient's hydration status a nurse would initiate:

A. Providing a variety of fluids
B. 7 classes of ice chips
C. Give fluids on patient demands
D. Maintain an intake and output chart

147. The nursing diagnosis, a nurse would frame in case of history of respiratory acidosis is:

A. Anxiety related to stress
B. Ineffective breathing pattern related to hyperventilation
C. Impaired gas exchange related to inadequate ventilation
D. High risk for injury related to nervous system excitability

---

141 A 142 C 143 C 144 C 145 D 146 D 147 C

148. **A direct intravenous infusion of this drug is fatal:**
A. Sodium bi-carbonate
B. Potassium chloride
C. Calcium
D. Atropine

149. **Each milliliter of fluid contains:**
A. 60 micro drops
B. 50 micro drops
C. 40 micro drops
D. 30 micro drops

150. **Each milliliter of fluid makes:**
A. 15 macro drops
B. 40 macro drops
C. 30 macro drops
D. 10 macro drops

151. **Each macro drop consist of:**
A. 4 micro drops
B. 5 micro drops
C. 3 micro drops
D. 6 micro drops

152. **One ounce of fluid contains:**
A. 30 ml
B. 40 ml
C. 50 ml
D. 60 ml

153. **The most important factor in providing culturally sensitive nursing care is:**
A. Communication
B. Time orientation
C. Biological variation
D. Environmental control

154. **Healthcare treatment is discouraged on a holy day by:**
A. Islam
B. Hinduism
C. Buddism
D. Christianity

155. **For Hindus it is important for a nurse to consider:**
A. Some sects are vegetarians
B. Followers must observed fast days
C. Many individuals avoid meals
D. Members abstain from alcohol

156. **The measurable aspect of a person's increase in physical dimension:**
A. Growth
B. Development
C. Maturation
D. Growth and development

---

148 B 149 A 150 A 151 A 152 A 153 A 154 C
155 A 156 A

157. The behavioural aspect of a person's adaptation to the environment is:
A. Growth
B. Development
C. Maturation
D. Growth and development

158. The biological plan for growth and development is:
A. Growth
B. Development
C. Maturation
D. Growth and development

159. A nurse need to tell the parents of a pre-schooler that a major cause of mortality of this child is:
A. Violence
B. Poison
C. Infectious diseases
D. Motor vehicle accidents

160. Health education for young adults to be related to the activities of:
A. Health promotion
B. Primary prevention
C. Secondary prevention
D. Tertiary prevention

161. Women should increase their daily calcium intake to 1000 to 1500 mg to prevent:
A. Arthritis
B. Osteoporosis
C. Hypertension
D. Coronary artery diseases

162. Initiative verses guild psychosocial development occurs in the:
A. Pre-schooler
B. Infant
C. Child-hood
D. Toddler

163. Industry verses inferiority psychosocial development occurs in the:
A. Pre-schooler
B. Infant
C. Childhood
D. Toddler

164. Identity verses identity diffusion psychosocial development occurs in the:
A. Adolescence
B. Infant
C. Childhood
D. Toddler

---

157 B 158 C 159 D 160 A 161 B 162 A 163 C
164 A

165. **Autonomy verses shame and doubt psychosocial development occurs in the:**
   A. Adolescence B. Infant
   C. Childhood D. Toddler

166. **Trust verses mistrust psychosocial development occurs in the:**
   A. Adolescence B. Infant
   C. Childhood D. Toddler

167. **Toddlers often participate in:**
   A. Parallel play B. Solitary play
   C. Non-associative play D. Opposite sex play

168. **The onset of menstruation is the:**
   A. Menarche B. Puberty
   C. Menopause D. Maturation

169. **The term used to describe the decline of the reproductive capacity and accompanying changes brought about by the decrease in sexual hormones is:**
   A. Climacteric B. Menopause
   C. Depression D. Regression

170. **The disorder that affect older adult's memory and cognitive function is the:**
   A. Dementia B. Insomnia
   C. Aphasia D. Dyspepsia

171. **Disturbed language disorder is termed as:**
   A. Dementia B. Insomnia
   C. Aphasia D. Dyspepsia

172. **Impaired motor activity is known as:**
   A. Dementia B. Insomnia
   C. Aphasia D. Apraxia

173. **The inability to recognize objects is called:**
   A. Dementia B. Insomnia
   C. Aphasia D. Agnosia

---

165 D 166 B 167 A 168 A 169 A 170 A 171 C
172 D 173 D

174. Which one represents people view themselves ?
A. Self concept
B. Self esteem
C. Self realize
D. Self identity

175. Emotional evaluation of self worth is the:
A. Self concept
B. Self esteem
C. Self realize
D. Self identity

176. The components of self concept is the following *except:*
A. Self esteem
B. Body image
C. Role
D. Behaviour

177. A person's clear persistent preference for another person of one sex or the other is known as:
A. Sexual response
B. Sexual behaviour
C. Sexual preference
D. Sexual orientation

178. Inability or difficulty in sexual functioning caused by physiological or psychological factors or both is called:
A. Sexual behaviour
B. Sexual response
C. Sexual orientation
D. Sexual dysfunction

179. Gender identity is the individual's:
A. Sense of being masculine
B. Sense of preferring one sex over the other
C. Sense of sexual behaviour
D. Sense of having sexual orientation

180. The family includes relatives in addition to the nuclear family is:
A. Joint family
B. Extended family
C. Blended family
D. Single parent family

181. The family formed when one parent leaves the nuclear family is:
A. Joint family
B. Extended family
C. Blended family
D. Single parent family

---

174 A 175 B 176 D 177 D 178 D 179 B 180 B
181 D

182. The family formed when parents bring unrelated children is:
A. Joint family
B. Extended family
C. Blended family
D. Single parent family

183. Family functioning involves:
A. The process used by the family to achieve goals
B. The patterns of people who are considered to be family members
C. The ongoing membership of the family
D. The pattern of relationships

184. Family structure is:
A. The process used by the family to achieve goals
B. The patterns of people who are considered to be family members
C. The ongoing membership of the family and the pattern of relationships
D. Intra familiar system of support

185. Family assessment includes:
A. Assessing individual family members separately
B. Assessing only those members living in the household
C. Assessing only the patient's perception of family interaction
D. Assessing individual family member and their interaction with one another and the patient

186. When planning care for the family a nurse need to:
A. Consider the developmental stage of the family
B. Include only the ill family members
C. Understand that the family will always help
D. Understand the cultural background is an important factor

187. When working with a family with a rigid family structure, interventions are designed to:
A. Attempt to change the family structure
B. Include only the most flexible family members
C. Create interventions that require minimal change
D. Provide solutions for problems only when they arise

---

182 C 183 A 184 C 185 D 186 D 187 A

188. **While assessing a person for effects of the general adaptation syndrome, a nurse should be aware that:**
   A. Heart rate increases in the resistance stage
   B. Blood volume increases in the exhaustion stage
   C. Vital signs returns to normal in the exhaustion stage
   D. Blood glucose level increases during the alarm reaction stage

189. **While teaching a person with hypertension about how stress can cause illness, a nurse explain that:**
   A. Hypertension causes stress by suppressing immunity
   B. Some anti-hypertensive drugs cause stress and illness
   C. A person on anti-hypertensive treatment has an immunity to stress
   D. Stress may cause a person to forget to take medication and thereby cause illness

190. **Any loss of a person or object that can no longer be felt, heard, known or experienced by the individual is:**
   A. Actual loss
   B. Perceived loss
   C. Maturational loss
   D. Situational loss

191. **Any loss, i.e. tangible and uniquely defined by the grieving patient is:**
   A. Actual loss
   B. Perceived loss
   C. Maturational loss
   D. Situational loss

192. **Any change in the developmental process, i.e. normally expected during a life time is:**
   A. Actual loss
   B. Perceived loss
   C. Maturational loss
   D. Situational loss

193. **Any sudden, unexpected external event, i.e. not predictable is:**
   A. Actual loss
   B. Perceived loss
   C. Maturational loss
   D. Situational loss

---

188 D 189 D 190 A 191 B 192 C 193 D

194. The stage in which an individual acts as though nothing has happened and may refuse to believe or understand that a loss has occurred is:
A. Denial
B. Anger
C. Bargaining
D. Depression

195. The stage in which the individual resist the loss and may strike out at everyone and everything is:
A. Denial
B. Anger
C. Bargaining
D. Depression

196. The stage in which the individual postpones awareness after reality of the loss and may try to deal in a subtle or overt way as though the loss can be prevented is:
A. Denial
B. Anger
C. Bargaining
D. Depression

197. The stage in which a person finally realizes the full impact and significance of the loss is:
A. Denial
B. Anger
C. Bargaining
D. Depression

198. The stage in which the individual accepts the loss and begins to look to the future is:
A. Denial
B. Anger
C. Bargaining
D. Acceptance

199. The process of disengaging or letting go that occurs before an actual loss or death has occurred is called:
A. Anticipatory grief
B. Bereavement
C. Bargaining
D. Acceptance

200. The state of thought, feeling and activity that follows loss is:
A. Anticipatory grief
B. Bereavement
C. Bargaining
D. Acceptance

194 A 195 B 196 C 197 D 198 D 199 A 200 B

201. An anticipation of a continued good, an improvement or lessening of something unpleasant is:
A. Hope
B. Stress
C. Grief
D. Loss

202. A factor that uniquely influences an older adult's grief response is:
A. Cultural background
B. Social economic resources
C. Sense of contributions in life
D. Support available from family members

203. An example of a quality improvement outcome indicated is the:
A. Rate of post operative wound infection
B. Counting of narcotics by nurses
C. Number of patients receiving education
D. Time taken to transport patient from emergency to general ward

204. To prevent injury for a patient who begins to back during ambulation a nurse should:
A. Call for assistance
B. Slight down the patient's body to the floor
C. Instruct the client to sit on a nearest chair
D. Contact the person

205. A principle of good body mechanics includes:
A. Keeping knees in locked position
B. Maintaining a wide base of support
C. Bending at the knee to maintain gravity
D. Holding objects away from the body

206. Passive range of motion exercises prevent:
A. Contracture
B. Osteoporosis
C. Muscle atrophy
D. Renal calculi

---

201 A 202 C 203 A 204 B 205 B 206 A

207. A necessary safety precaution when ambulating a patient is to:
A. Have family members
B. Have patient to wear well fitting chapels/shoes
C. Have at least two people
D. Be sure pain medication was given

208. The equipment that would work best to help ambulate an unsteady patient is:
A. A walker
B. Crutches
C. Wheel chair
D. Mechanical lift device

209. A device that helps prevent foot drop is the:
A. Foot role
B. Foot board
C. Trochanter role
D. Ankle foot splints

210. To prevent a confused patient pulling at an IV line during hospitalization, the best nursing intervention is to:
A. Use an arm board
B. Apply wrist restraints
C. Put the side rails
D. Provide close observation of the patient

211. The first action a nurse should do on observation of an electrical fire in a patient's room is to:
A. Activate the fire alarm
B. Evacuate all patients
C. Confine the fire by closing all doors and windows
D. Extinguish the fire by using the nearest fire extinguisher

212. Initial intervention for a patient wandering in the hall looking for the bathroom during the night shift is to:
A. Insert a urinary catheter
B. Assign a staff member to stay with a patient
C. Ask the physician to order restraints
D. Provide scheduled toileting during the night shift

207 B 208 A 209 B 210 D 211 A 212 D

213. In planning care for the older adult patient trying to climb over the bed's side rails a nurse know that:
A. Older adults tolerate restraints well
B. Older adults must be restraint
C. Nurse is legally liable if she fail to restrain a confused older adult
D. Older adults are prone to confusion because of heightened sensitivity to medication

214. The restrain that is most restrictive for the patient that provides the least moment is:
A. The mitten
B. The west
C. Bylateral wrist restraint
D. Four bed side in the up-position

215. A medical/surgical unit decides to institute a fall prevention programme. A nurse know that:
A. Falls are difficult to prevent
B. All patients are at high risk for falling
C. A fractured hip is the most common injury after a fall
D. Older adults are more likely to fall because of a physiological changes of aging

216. When teaching parents about accidental poisoning in children, a nurse would instruct them to:
A. Give oral fluids
B. Induce vomiting
C. Call the poison control centre
D. Drive the child to the emergency department

217. When providing discharge teaching about homes safety to older patient, a nurse know that:
A. A safe environment promotes patient independence
B. Most accidents in the older adult are related to lifestyle factors
C. Older patients are reluctant to make necessary environmental changes
D. Environmental hazards are costly for the older adult on a fixed income

---

213 D 214 C 215 D 216 C 217 A

218. Key elements that place a patient at a greater risk for falls include:
A. History of falls, urinary frequency, smoking
B. History of falls, confusion, impaired mobility
C. History of falls, age over 60, seizure disorders
D. History of falls, sensory impairment, age over 60

219. In planning discharge teaching aimed at reducing safety risk in the home, a nurse recognize that:
A. Safety risk change in each developmental level
B. Patients are able to identify what their safety risk are
C. Assessment should focus on environmental factor
D. Teaching the patient and family about home safety is difficult to do in a hospital setting

220. During the first post-operative day following abdominal surgery the patient will probably require a:
A. Shower
B. Tub bath
C. Partial bath
D. Complete bed bath

221. In addition to bathing the following intervention may best assist in promoting patient comfort is:
A. Back rub
B. Books on tape
C. Night time snack
D. Mouth wash

222. The most important priority when providing oral hygiene to the unconscious patient is to:
A. Prevent aspiration
B. Prevent mouth odour
C. Prevent dental caries
D. Prevent mouth ulcers

223. The goal of meticulous foot care for patient is to:
A. Prevent injury to the dorsum of the feet
B. Provide routine cleaning of the feet and nails
C. Monitor the healing process of foot ulcers
D. Determine if the patients shoes are of the proper size

---

218 C 219 A 220 D 221 A 222 A 223 A

224. The method for trimming toe nails is to:
A. Cut the nail in a curve
B. Cut the nail straight across
C. Cut the nail toward the cuticles
D. Cut the nail to meet the safety of the finger

225. When providing hygiene to the older adult it is important to remember that the older adult's skin is:
A. Fragile with decreased elasticity
B. Fragile with increased elasticity
C. Fragile with increased circulation
D. Fragile with increased muscle mass

226. Bad breath from mouth is known as:
A. Halitosis
B. Cheilosis
C. Stomatitis
D. Gingivitis

227. Receding gum lines, inflammation, gaps between teeth is:
A. Halitosis
B. Cheilosis
C. Periodontitis
D. Gingivitis

228. Cracking of lips is known as:
A. Halitosis
B. Cheilosis
C. Stomatitis
D. Gingivitis

229. Inflammation of the mouth is known as:
A. Halitosis
B. Cheilosis
C. Stomatitis
D. Gingivitis

230. Inflammation of gum is known as:
A. Halitosis
B. Cheilosis
C. Stomatitis
D. Gingivitis

231. Risk factors for cardiopulmonary disease include:
A. Lack of exercise and poor nutrition
B. Family history of cough disease
C. Family history of smoking and obesity
D. Age, gender lack of exercise, high fat diet and obesity

---

224 B 225 A 226 A 227 C 228 B 229 C 230 D
231 D

232. Assessment of patient with tachycardia should include:
A. Risk factors for heart disease
B. Consumption of caffeine and herbal substances
C. Heart rate, blood pressure and respiratory rate
D. Nutritional assessment for high fat diet

233. When assessing the patients oxygenation a nurse would include:
A. Complete blood count and chest X-ray
B. Heart rate and respiratory rate
C. Arterial blood gases and pulse oximetry
D. Chest X-ray, heart rate, respiratory rate and arterial blood gases

234. The most reliable physical assessment indicator of low oxygen in the blood is:
A. Cyanosis
B. Increased heart rate
C. Increased blood pressure
D. Cyanosis of the oral mucosa or conjunctiva

235. A normal appearing electro-cardiogram tracing with a heart rate of 125 beats/minute would be considered as:
A. Sinus rhythm
B. Sinus bradycardia
C. Sinus tachycardia
D. Ventricular tachycardia

236. Incentive spirometry is used to:
A. Promote coughing
B. Replace the need for early ambulation
C. Increased deep breathing and prevent atelectasis
D. Keep the patient occupied post-operative

237. More precise oxygen concentration can be achieved using a:
A. Nasal cannula
B. Simple face mask
C. Venturi mask system
D. Plastic face mask

---

232 B 233 C 234 D 235 C 236 C 237 C

238. **In carrying the patient with multiple rib fracture a nurse must keep in mind that:**
    A. A tight rib binder will reduce pain
    B. Pain medication should be administered every 4 hours
    C. Deep breathing should not be implemented
    D. Impaired chest wall movement reduces the level of tissue oxygenation

239. **When carrying a patient with a decreased hemoglobin level it is important to remember that:**
    A. The patient is at risk for bleeding
    B. The patient has altered oxygen transport
    C. The patient is at risk for elevator CO_2 level
    D. The patient has alteration in the chemical regulators of respiration

240. **Restlessness, anxiety, decreased ability to concentrate, tachycardia and elevated blood pressure indicate:**
    A. Hypoxia
    B. Hypoxaemia
    C. Right sided heart failure
    D. Pulmonary diseases

241. **Contractions of the myocardium occurs:**
    A. Before the electrical activity
    B. During the electrical activity
    C. After the electrical activity
    D. None of the above

242. **Nurse should remember that a diastolic blood pressure in children is determined by:**
    A. At 45 mm Hg
    B. At 30 mm Hg
    C. Loss of sound
    D. When the sound becomes muffled

243. **Patients are candidates for chest physiotherapy if:**
    A. The patient is receiving long term steroids
    B. The patient has had abdominal surgery
    C. The patient has increased intracranial pressure
    D. The patient has good exercise tolerance and can follow instructions

---

238 D 239 B 240 A 241 C 242 D 243 D

244. A recurrent, altered state of consciousness that occurs for sustained period is known as:
A. Sleep
B. Insomnia
C. Sleep apnea
D. Narcolepsy

245. A symptom experience by patient who have chronic difficulty falling asleep, frequent awakenings from sleep and/ or a short sleep or non-restorative sleep is:
A. Sleep
B. Insomnia
C. Sleep apnea
D. Narcolepsy

246. A disorder in which the individual cannot breathe and sleep at the same time is:
A. Sleep
B. Insomnia
C. Sleep apnea
D. Narcolepsy

247. A CNS disfunction of mechanisms that regulate sleep and wake state is:
A. Sleep
B. Insomnia
C. Sleep apnea
D. Narcolepsy

248. A problem many patients have as a result of the dyssomnias is:
A. Sleep
B. Insomnia
C. Sleep apnea
D. Sleep deprivation

249. Sleep disorders that produce undesirable physical symptoms as a result of autonomic nervous system changes and skeletal muscle activity during sleep are:
A. Sleep
B. Insomnia
C. Sleep apnea
D. Parasomnias

250. Tooth grinding is otherwise known as:
A. Sleep
B. Sleep bruxism
C. Sleep apnea
D. Narcolepsy

251. The most common symptom reported by a patient for obstructive sleep apnea is:
A. Headache
B. Early wakening
C. Impaired reasoning
D. Excessive daytime sleep

---

244 A 245 B 246 C 247 D 248 D 249 D 250 B
251 D

252. **Sleeping medication should not be prescribed for longer than:**
   A. 1 week
   B. 2 weeks
   C. 2-3 weeks
   D. 4-5 weeks

253. **A priority nursing intervention to promote sleep in the hospitalized patient is to:**
   A. Turn TV on low to late night programming
   B. Finish all the laboratory investigation by 5 pm
   C. Give patient sleeping medication by 11 pm
   D. Encourage to continue to follow regular bedtime routines

254. **A priority nursing goal for an older patient compliance about difficulty in falling asleep is to:**
   A. Sleep for 7 hours each night
   B. Limit nappin during the day to 3 or 4
   C. Decreased awakenings to 2 or 3 at night
   D. Fall asleep within 20 minutes of getting in bed

255. **Nurse explained to a patient that the most vivid dreaming occurs during:**
   A. REM sleep
   B. Stage-I NREM sleep
   C. Stage-IV NREM sleep
   D. Transition from NREM to REM sleep

256. **Beta-adrenergic blockers taking by patient for hypertension may interfere with normal sleep patterns by:**
   A. Causing nocturia
   B. Increasing daytime sleep
   C. Causing awakenings from sleep
   D. Increasing difficulty in falling asleep

257. **An intervention to include on a care plan for an older patient who is having difficulty in sleeping is to:**
   A. Nap during the day
   B. Exercise in the evening
   C. Allow the patient to sleep as late as possible
   D. Decreased fluids 2-4 hours before going to bed

---

252 C 253 D 254 D 255 A 256 C 257 D

258. A nursing measure to promote sleep in young children is to:
A. Make sure the room is dark and quite
B. Allow children to fall asleep in parent's bed
C. Increase evening activities
D. Encourage reading a story just before bedtime

259. The question a nurse ask to a mother having three-year-old boy having sleep problems is:
A. The age of other siblings in the home
B. Usual bedtime practices for the child
C. Growth and development patterns for the child
D. The type of preschool the child attends during the day

260. One of the reasons that many nurses avoid acknowledging a patient's pain is:
A. Inadequate pain management skills
B. Insufficient time to respond to the patient
C. Fear that the drug may cause addiction
D. Inability to manage the increased patient load

261. Nursing intervention for a 82-year-old patient with Alzheimer's disease who is restless and moaning and did not sleep well most of the night is to:
A. Restrain the patient
B. Obtain a psychiatric consultation
C. Administer Tylenor two tablets by mouth
D. Assess and document physical and behavioural activities

262. When carrying for a patient with cancer pain, a nurse should:
A. Begin with opioids to ensure pain relief
B. Administer pain medication with caution
C. Be administer lower doses of opioids
D. Begin with higher doses of prescribed medication

263. 30 minutes after a heat therapy on wake massage, a nurse should:
A. Turn and reposition the patient
B. Document the care
C. Evaluate the effects of the therapy
D. Administer the prescribed pain reliever

---

258 D 259 B 260 C 261 D 262 D 263 C

264. A preventive approach for acute pain relief means that analgesic medications are given:
A. Before the pain is experienced
B. With complimentary therapies
C. Before the pain becomes severe
D. When the pain tolerance level is exceeded

265. Positive nitrogen balance would occur in:
A. Infection
B. Starvation
C. Burns
D. Pregnancy

266. The nutrient that provides the body's most preferred energy source is:
A. Fat
B. Protein
C. Vitamin
D. Carbohydrate

267. The nutrient that is preferred to repair tissue is:
A. Fat
B. Protein
C. Vitamin
D. Carbohydrate

268. When feeding tubes are first position, verification is done by:
A. Auscultation
B. X-ray
C. pH testing
D. Confirmation of distal mark on the tube

269. The most accurate method for bedside confirmation of feeding tube placement is:
A. Auscultation
B. X-ray
C. pH testing
D. Confirmation of distal mark on the tube

270. Parenteral nutrition is used when the patient is:
A. Nil per oral
B. Critically ill
C. Recovery from abdominal surgery
D. Experiencing gastrointestinal disfunction

---

264 C 265 D 266 D 267 B 268 B 269 C 270 D

271. Assessment of glucose balance in a patient on parenteral nutrition is most accurate with:
A. Fasting blood glucose
B. Urine test for acetone
C. Urine test for glucose
D. Serum glucose monitoring

272. Ideal weight loss for an over weight patient to achieve weight reduction is:
A. 1 kg per week
B. 1-2 kg per week
C. 2-3 kg per week
D. More than 3 kg per week

273. Initial action for an adult patient who has not voided for 12 hours and have urge to pass urine is to:
A. Notify the physician
B. Insert a catheter
C. Palpate the patient bladder
D. Increase fluid intake

274. Identification of a two plus haematuria in female patient with a urinary tract infection indicates:
A. A response to the antibiotic therapy
B. A ruptured vessel within the bladder
C. Irritation of the bladder mucosa from the pathogen
D. The result of a straight catheter used to obtain a sterile specimen

275. First action for a patient who underwent bladder surgery having bright red urine in his catheter drainage bag is to:
A. Notify the physician
B. Obtain patients vital sign
C. Irrigate the catheter
D. Monitor the vital sign every 15 minutes till physician comes

276. When applying a condom catheter, it is important to secure the catheter to the penile shaft in such a manner that the:
A. Catheter is tight and drain in well
B. Catheter is dependent and draining well
C. Catheter is secured with adhesive tape applied in a circular pattern
D. Catheter is snug and secure but does not cause constriction to blood flow

---

271 D 272 A 273 C 274 C 275 B 276 D

277. **Patient with urinary track infection experience:**
   A. Only pain on urination
   B. Decreased frequency, burning and pain
   C. Increased frequency, hesitancy and pain
   D. Increased frequency, hesitancy, burning and pain on urination

278. **Maintaining a foley catheter drainage bag in the dependent position prevents:**
   A. Urinary reflux
   B. Urinary retention
   C. Reflex incontinence
   D. Urinary incontinence

279. **The purpose of instructing the patient to begin and discard the initial stream of urine when obtaining a mid-stream urine specimen is to:**
   A. Allow for patient comfort
   B. Allow sufficient urine to be obtained for the culture specimen
   C. Allow the initial urine to wash bacteria from the external genitalia
   D. Allow the initial urine to drain from the bladder to avoid in accurate urine culture

280. **Hospital acquired urine tract infection are called:**
   A. Viral
   B. Fungal
   C. Bacterial
   D. Nosocomial

281. **Hospital acquired urinary tract infection are most frequently caused by inadequate hand washing and:**
   A. Urinary drainage bags
   B. Poor perineal hygiene
   C. Catheterization procedure
   D. Poor hand washing technique

282. **Most nutrients and electrolytes are absorbed in the:**
   A. Colon B. Stomach
   C. Oesophagus D. Small intestine

277 D 278 A 279 C 280 D 281 D 282 D

283. A nurse will instruct the 55-year-old patient come for a routine physical check-up to obtain a fecal occult blood specimen:
A. When there is a family history of polyps
B. If patient reports rectal bleeding
C. If a palpable mass is detected on digital examination
D. As a part of a routine examination

284. Diarrhea that occurs with a fecal impaction is the result of:
A. A clear liquid diet
B. Irritation of the intestinal mucosa
C. Seepage of stool around the impaction
D. Inability of the patient to form a stool

285. To determine the cause of periostomal irritation by a ostomate a nurse must assess:
A. Circulation to stoma and fit of pouch
B. Quantity and consistency of fecal drainage in the pouch
C. Presence of signs of infection at the stoma
D. Circulation to stoma, allergic response to ostomy product, etc

286. The maximum amount given for a 55 year old patient to whom a cleansing enema is ordered:
A. 150-200 ml
B. 200-400 ml
C. 400-750 ml
D. 750-1000 ml

287. Action to be taken for a patient who have blood in the return fluid and rectal bleeding following enema is:
A. Stop the instillation
B. Slow down the rate of instillation
C. Stop the instillation and obtain vital sign
D. Tell the patient to breathe slowly

288. A physiological risk associated with prolonged immobility is:
A. Decreased bone resorption
B. Increased cardiac work-load
C. Decreased serum calcium levels
D. Increased hemoglobin formation

---

283 C 284 C 285 D 286 D 287 C 288 B

289. **The most important objective of bed rest for a patient with bilateral pneumonia would be to:**
   A. Allow the patient uninterrupted sleep
   B. Reduce the oxygen needs of the body
   C. Decrease the need for pain medication
   D. Prevent the patient from falling

290. **Dropping of systolic blood pressure when making the patient to stand after several days of bed rest is referred as:**
   A. Rebound hypotension
   B. Orthostatic hypotension
   C. Positional hypotension
   D. Central venous hypotension

291. **A nursing diagnosis related to the safety of the patient who has been helped to get out of bed after 5 days of immobilization because of extensive abdominal surgery would be:**
   A. Pain
   B. Impaired skin integrity
   C. Risk for activity in tolerance
   D. Altered tissue perfusion

292. **The purpose of elastic stockings after a surgical procedure is to:**
   A. Prevent varicose veins
   B. Prevent muscular atrophy
   C. Ensure joint mobility and prevent contractures
   D. Facilitate the return of venous blood to the heart

293. **The priority intervention for a patient to whom a nurse suspect a deep vein thrombosis in the left lower leg is:**
   A. Check for homan's sign immediately
   B. Massage the area to promote circulation
   C. Prepare the patient for radiological studies
   D. Apply elastic stockings

---

289 B 290 B 291 C 292 D 293 C

294. A priority nursing intervention for a patient who have a past history of chronic obstructive pulmonary disease and advice one week bed rest for fracture hip is:
A. Increased fluid intake
B. Perform leg exercises every hour
C. Perform incentive spirometry every hour while awake
D. Ask for pain medication at a very onset of discomfort

295. Nursing intervention for a patient to whom a nurse suspect pulmonary emboli is to:
A. Call the physician immediately
B. Place the patient in fowler's position and assess oxygenation status
C. Encourage the patient to take deep breath to promote lung expansion
D. Place the patient in a supine position to prevent dislodgement of the clot

296. The patient at greatest risk for developing adverse effects of immobility is a:
A. Three-year-old with a fractured femur
B. 40-year-old woman following thyroidectomy
C. 78-year-old man in traction for a broken hip
D. 30-year-old woman undergoing a hysterectomy

297. The red spot blanches with fingertip pressure over a bony prominence on an immobile patient indicates:
A. A local skin infection
B. Sensitive skin
C. A stage III pressure ulcer
D. Blanching hyperemia reaction that causes the blood vessels to dilate

298. Pressure injury to the skin results from:
A. Blood vessel damage to repeated infections
B. Continual exposure of the skin to fecal or urinary incontinence
C. Skin compressed by two surfaces for a prolonged period of time
D. Excessive dryness of the epidermis

294 C 295 B 296 C 297 D 298 C

299. The topical management of a clean granular wound healing by secondary intension requires:

A. A moist wound dressing
B. An antibiotic cream application
C. Whirlpool treatments to stimulate granulation tissue
D. Exposure of the wound to air twice a day

300. The specimen for culture from a wound should be taken from:

A. The necrotic tissue
B. The wound drainage
C. The drainage on the dressing
D. Clean healthy looking tissue

301. Serous drainage from a wound is defined as:

A. Fresh bleeding
B. Thick and yellow
C. Clear watery plasma
D. Beige to brown and foul smelling

302. Interventions to manage a patient with fecal and urinary incontinence includes:

A. Use of a large absorbent diaper
B. Keeping the buttocks expose to air
C. Use of an incontinence cleanser followed by application of a moisture barrier ointment
D. Frequent cleansing, application of an ointment and covering the area with a thick absorbent towel

303. The best description of a hydrocolloid dressing is:

A. A seaweed derivative that is highly absorptive
B. Premoistured gauze placed over a granulating wound
C. A debriding enzyme that is used to remove necrotic tissue
D. A dressing that forms a gel that interacts with the wound surface

304. A binder placed around a surgical patient with a new abdominal wound is indicated for:

A. Collection of wound drainage
B. Reduction of abdominal swelling
C. Reduction of stress on the abdominal incision
D. Stimulation of peristalsis from direct pressure

---

299 A 300 D 301 C 302 C 303 D 304 C

305. Application of a warm compress is indicated:
A. To relieve oedema
B. For a patient who is shivering
C. To promote healing by stimulating blood flow
D. To protect bony prominences from pressure ulcers

306. The older adult under normal physiological changes experience include:
A. Decreased sensitivity to glare
B. Increased number of taste buds
C. Increased peripheral neuropathy
D. Difficulty in discriminating vowel sounds

307. Common side effects of non-steroidal anti-inflammatory drugs include:
A. Ototoxicity
B. Loss of taste
C. Optic irritation
D. Alternation in vision

308. For a hearing impaired patient to better hear a spoken conversation, a nurse should:
A. Approach the patient quietly from behind
B. Use a louder tone of voice
C. Select a public area to have a spoken conversation
D. Use her hands and eyes as visual aids while speaking

309. When obtaining a history of the patient's hearing loss, a nurse should ask:
A. How long have you been deaf ?
B. Do you also have vision problems ?
C. Why don't you pay attention to me ?
D. How does your hearing loss compare to a year ago ?

310. An intervention to properly introduce stimuli for a hospitalized patient who is disoriented would be to:
A. Keep the room darken
B. Introduce an all talk radio programme
C. Speak with the patient in muted tones
D. Draw back dividing curtains

305 A 306 C 307 A 308 D 309 D 310 D

311. The assessment data that best indicates signs of sensory deprivation include:

A. Deminished anxiety
B. Altered spatial perception
C. Improved completion of task
D. Decreased need for physical stimulation

312. A realistic goal for an older adult driving patient is to:

A. Drive very very slowly all of the time
B. Keep the car in good working condition
C. Always drive at night to prevent sun glare
D. Drive during rush hours when others are on the road

313. An intervention a nurse include in teaching parents of hearing impaired children is to:

A. Avoid activities in which crowds and loud noises occur
B. Delay childhood immunization
C. Take precautions when involved in activities associated with high intensity noises
D. Prophylactically administer antibiotics to reduce the incidence of infections

314. An intervention a nurse will make for a poorly illuminated patient's environment is by:

A. Using fluorescent lightening
B. Recommending muted colours
C. Doubling the amount of light
D. Placing incandescent higher voltage light bulbs into light fixtures

315. A high priority home assessment for a patient with diminished olfaction is the inclusion of:

A. Low water heater setting
B. Extra lighting in hall
C. Smoke detectors on all levels
D. Amplified telephone receivers

---

311 B 312 B 313 C 314 D 315 C

316. As a result of sensory deficits the patient may:
- A. Rely solely on one sense
- B. Respond normally to stimuli
- C. Withdrawn socially to hope with the loss
- D. Function safely within their environment

317. When assessing for the effects of a sensory deprivation a nurse should be aware that the patient will demonstrate:
- A. Calm demeanor
- B. Normal behaviour
- C. Deminished level of anxiety
- D. Difficulty with problem solving

318. An obese patient is at risk for poor wound healing post-operatively because:
- A. Ventilatory capacity is reduced
- B. Fatty tissue has a poor blood supply
- C. Risk for dehiscence is increased
- D. Resuming normal, physical activity is delayed

319. Because an older adult is at increased risk for respiratory complication after surgery, a nurse must:
- A. Ambulate patient every 2 hours
- B. Monitor fluid and electrolyte status every shift
- C. Orient the patient to surrounding environment
- D. Encourage the patient to turn, deep breathe and cough frequently

320. Pre-operatively a nurse collect the history of all drugs taken because they:
- A. May cause allergies to develop
- B. May interact with anaesthetic agents
- C. Will need to be reordered after surgery
- D. Should be taken in the morning of surgery day with water

321. A patient with increased prothrombing time or an activated partial thrompoplastine time is at risk post-operatively for:
- A. Anaemia
- B. Bleeding
- C. Infection
- D. Cardiac disorders

316 C 317 D 318 B 319 D 320 B 321 B

322. **A patient who smokes two packs of cigarettes per day is most at risk post-operatively for:**
   A. Infection
   B. Pneumonia
   C. Hypotension
   D. Drug withdrawal

323. **When monitoring pain post-operatively a nurse must ask patient if he is experiencing pain and document:**
   A. The patients pain scale rating
   B. The patients level of consciousness
   C. What the patients wants for treatment
   D. How often the patient asks for pain medication

324. **The fluid balance is best monitored by:**
   A. Skin turger
   B. Daily weight
   C. Capillary refill
   D. Intake and output

325. **A patient on the first post-operative day is at risk for hemorrhage. A nurse should always:**
   A. Turn the patient to check underneath
   B. Reinforce a dry dressing to add more padding
   C. Have the patient used a pillow to splint the incision
   D. Remove the dressing to look directly at the incision

326. **The action the nurse would take for a patient who is having dyspnea, because often instruction is:**
   A. Suction the pharynx and bronchial tree
   B. Give oxygen through mask at 10 litre/minute
   C. Position the patient so that the tongue falls forward
   D. Ask the patient to use an incentive spirometer

327. **Early ambulation is ordered post operatively to prevent the post-operative complication of:**
   A. Pain
   B. Nausea
   C. Wound dehiscence
   D. Deep vein thrombosis

---

322 B 323 A 324 B 325 A 326 C 327 D

328. Family members to be included when a nurse teach the patient pre-operative exercises show that the time:

A. Supervise the patient at home
B. Coach the patient post-operatively
C. Practice with the patient while waiting for surgery
D. Relieve the nurse by get-in the patient to do exercises

329. Sitting position is the best position for doing deep breathing and coughing exercises, because this position:

A. Is more comfortable
B. Facilitates expansion of the thorax
C. Increases the patients view of the room
D. Help the patient to splint with a pillow

330. Reason for doing leg exercises during post-operatively is to:

A. Decrease leg fatigue
B. Increase muscle tone
C. Increase venous return
D. Maintain blood pressure

331. Movement of a limp away from the body is:

A. Abduction
B. Adduction
C. Fluxion
D. Exemption

332. Movement of a limp toward the body is:

A. Abduction
B. Adduction
C. Fluxion
D. Exemption

333. Partial or complete loss of hair is:

A. Alopecia
B. Aphasia
C. Agnosea
D. Apnea

334. Lack or loss of appetite:

A. Alopecia
B. Anorexia
C. Agnosea
D. Apnea

---

328 B 329 B 330 C 331 A 332 B 333 A 334 B

335. **Defective or absent of language function is:**
A. Alopecia
B. Anorexia
C. Aphasia
D. Apnea

336. **Absence of germs or micro organisms is:**
A. Asepsis
B. Sepsis
C. Infection
D. Infestation

337. **Presence of bacteria in the urine is:**
A. Bacteriuria
B. Polyuria
C. Anuria
D. Haematuria

338. **Audible abdominal sounds produced by hyperactive intestinal peristalsis is:**
A. Borborygmus
B. Flatulence
C. Dympinitis
D. None of these

339. **Abnormal sound or murmur heard while auscultating an organ, gland or artery is:**
A. Bruit
B. Bruxism
C. Proporygmi
D. Buccal

340. **Condition characterized by sudden muscular weakness and loss of muscle tone is:**
A. Cataplexy
B. Autopsy
C. Narcoplexy
D. Biopsy

341. **Drugs that act to promote bowel evacuation is:**
A. Cathartics
B. Emetics
C. Suppository
D. Emollient

342. **Condition characterized by difficulty in passing stool or and infrequent passage of hard stool is:**
A. Constipation
B. Obstipation
C. Construction
D. Concentration

343. **Debridement is the removal of ______ from a wound:**
A. Death tissue
B. Purse
C. Dead skin
D. Any drainage

---

335 C 336 A 337 A 338 A 339 A 340 A 341 A
342 A 343 A

344. Secretion of sweat especially profuse secretion is:
A. Diaphoresis
B. Perspiration
C. Diffusion
D. Dehydration

345. Increase in the number of stools and the passage of liquid unformed feces is:
A. Diarrhea
B. Constipation
C. Fecal impaction
D. Obstipation

346. Painfull menstruation is:
A. Dysmenorrhea
B. Dysrhythmias
C. Dysuria
D. Diarrhea

347. Painfull urination is:
A. Dysmenorrhea
B. Dysrhythmias
C. Dysuria
D. Diarrhea

348. Absence of lens is:
A. Ectropion
B. Aphakia
C. Neuropion
D. Entorphia

349. Abnormal accumulation of fluid in interstitial spaces of tissues is:
A. Oedema
B. Sarcoma
C. Eczema
D. Erythema

350. Eversion of the eyelid inward toward the eye is:
A. Ectropion
B. Entropion
C. Neuropion
D. Entorphin

351. Normal respiration is:
A. Dyspnea
B. Apnea
C. Eupnea
D. Orthopnea

352. Accumulation of hardened fecal material in the rectum or sigmoid colon is:
A. Fecal impaction
B. Fecal incontinence
C. Constipation
D. Obstipation

---

344 A 345 A 346 A 347 C 348 B 349 A 350 B
351 C 352 A

353. **Inability to control passage of feces and gas from the anus is:**
   A. Fecal impaction
   B. Fecal incontinence
   C. Constipation
   D. Obstipation

354. **Vomiting of blood is:**
   A. Haematemesis
   B. Haemoptysis
   C. Epitaxis
   D. Melena

355. **Collection of blood dropped in the tissues after skin is:**
   A. Haematoma
   B. Haemoptysis
   C. Epitaxis
   D. Melena

356. **Abnormal presence of blood in the urine is:**
   A. Haematoma
   B. Haemoptysis
   C. Epitaxis
   D. Haematuria

357. **Coughing up of blood is:**
   A. Haematoma
   B. Haemoptysis
   C. Epitaxis
   D. Melena

358. **Greater than normal amounts of CO_2 in the blood is:**
   A. Hypercapnea
   B. Haemoptysis
   C. Epitaxis
   D. Melena

359. **Pneumonia that results from fluid accumulation as a result of inactivity is:**
   A. Hypostatic pneumonia
   B. Orthostatic pneumonia
   C. Aspirated pneumonia
   D. Bacterial pneumonia

360. **Infection caused by a treatment or diagnostic procedure is:**
   A. Iatrogenic infection
   B. Infection
   C. Acquired infection
   D. None of these

361. **Insertion of a breathing tube through the mouth or nose into the trachea to ensure a patient airway is:**
   A. Intubation
   B. Aspiration
   C. Ventilation
   D. None of these

---

353 B 354 A 355 A 356 D 357 B 358 A 359 A
360 A 361 A

362. **Sound heard during the taking of blood pressure using a sphygmomanometer is:**
A. Korotkoff sound B. Bruit sound
C. Visceral sound D. Vocal sound

363. **Drug that acts to promote bowel evacuation is:**
A. Laxative B. Purgative
C. Emolient D. Antihelmenthic

364. **Procedures used to reduce the number of micro-organisms and prevent their spread is:**
A. Medical asepsis B. Surgical asepsis
C. Antiseptic D. Sepsis

365. **Bleeding per rectum is:**
A. Melena B. Haematuria
C. Haematoma D. Haemorrhage

366. **Onset of a girl's first menstruation is:**
A. Menarche B. Menopause
C. Medicoid D. Micturition

367. **Uncontrolable desire to sleep that occur several times during a day is:**
A. Narcolepsy B. Nocturia
C. Biopsy D. Autopsy

368. **Urination at night is:**
A. Narcolepsy
B. Nocturia
C. Biopsy
D. Autopsy

369. **Infections acquired during hospitalization is:**
A. Nosocomial infection
B. Infestation
C. Iatrogenic infection
D. Infection

370. **Involuntary, rhythmical movements of the eyes is:**
A. Nystagmus B. Ptosis
C. Narcolepsy D. Biopsy

362 A 363 A 364 A 365 A 366 A 367 A 368 B
369 A 370 A

371. Surgical procedure in which an opening is made:
A. Ostomy B. Otomy
C. Raphy D. Autopsy

372. Temporary paralysis of intestinal wall is:
A. Paralytic ileus B. Peristalsis
C. Tympanitis D. Flatulence

373. Determining the density of a body part by striking of short sharp taps of the fingers is:
A. Percussion B. Palpation
C. Auscultation D. Inspection

374. Tiny purple or red spots that appear on skin is:
A. Petechiae B. Erythemia
C. Eczema D. Dermatitis

375. Presence of protein in the urine is:
A. Proteinuria B. Polyuria
C. Anuria D. Dysuria

376. Symptom of itching is:
A. Pruritus B. Dermatitis
C. Petechiae D. None of these

377. Condition in which the radial pulse is less than the ventricular rate is:
A. Pulse deficit B. Pulse pressure
C. Apical pulse D. Radial pulse

378. Difference between the systolic and diastolic pressure is:
A. Pulse deficit B. Pulse pressure
C. Apical pulse D. Radial pulse

379. Device to aid in the immobilization of a patient is:
A. Restrain B. Pillow
C. Bed blocks D. Heart rest

380. Bath in which only the hips or buttocks are immersed in fluid is:
A. Sitz bath B. Shower
C. Bed bath D. Bath

---

371 A 372 A 373 A 374 A 375 A 376 A 377 A
378 B 379 A 380 A

381. **Cessation of breathing for a time during sleep is:**
A. Sleep apnea
B. Sleep bradypnea
C. Dyspnea
D. Apnea

382. **Administration of medication underneath the patient's tongue is:**
A. Sublingual
B. Oral
C. Parental
D. None of these

383. **Secondary infection usually caused by an opportunistic pathogen is:**
A. Super infection
B. Nosocomial infection
C. Iatrogenic infection
D. Infestation

384. **Procedures used to eliminate any micro-organisms from any area is:**
A. Surgical asepsis
B. Medical asepsis
C. Sepsis
D. Antiseptic

385. **A brief lapse in consciousness caused by transient cerebral hypoxia is:**
A. Synapse
B. Syncope
C. Sympathy
D. Synergy

386. **Chemical or physiological agents that may produce adverse effects in the embryo or fetus is:**
A. Teratogens
B. Halogens
C. Collagens
D. Colloid

387. **Ringing heard in one or both ears is:**
A. Tinnitus
B. Nystagmus
C. Tympanitis
D. None of these

388. **Flora not commonly found in a particular area of the body is:**
A. Transcient flora
B. Resident flora
C. Normal flora
D. None of these

389. **A one that is used to prevent external rotation of the legs is:**
A. Trochanter roll
B. Hand roll
C. Pillow
D. Back rest

---

381 A 382 A 383 A 384 A 385 B 386 A 387 A
388 A 389 A

390. Inability to control urination is urinary:
A. Incontinence
B. Reflux
C. Retention
D. Diversion

391. Abnormal backward flow of urine is:
A. Incontinence
B. Reflux
C. Retention
D. Diversion

392. Sensation of dizziness or spinning is:
A. Vertigo
B. Syncop
C. Synapse
D. Synergy

393. Presence of pus in the urine is:
A. Pyuria
B. Anuria
C. Dysuria
D. Oliguria

394. Absence of urine is:
A. Pyuria
B. Anuria
C. Dysuria
D. Oliguria

395. Passing of urine below normal is:
A. Pyuria
B. Anuria
C. Dysuria
D. Oliguria

396. Crepitus is seen in:
A. Fracture
B. Bleeding
C. Vomiting
D. Wounds

397. Insomnia means:
A. Absence of sleep
B. Excessive sleep
C. Sleep hygiene
D. Sleep disturbance

398. Source of primary data is:
A. Medical record
B. Patient
C. Family members
D. Healthcare team

399. The safest position for an unconscious patient is:
A. Lateral
B. Prone
C. Supine
D. Dorsal

400. To prevent tongue falling back the safest position is:
A. Lateral
B. Prone
C. Supine
D. Dorsal

---

390 A 391 B 392 A 393 A 394 B 395 D 396 A
397 A 398 B 399 A 400 A

401. After surgery patient should void urine within:
A. 8 to10 hours
B. 10 to15 hours
C. 15 to 20 hours
D. 20 to 25 hours

402. After surgery patient being assisted from bed to sit on a chair for a short period within:
A. 12 hours
B. 18 hours
C. 24 hours
D. 36 hours

403. Difficulties in expression is the communication barrier of:
A. Physiological
B. Cultural
C. Psychological
D. Environmental

404. Emotional disturbance is the communication barrier of:
A. Physiological
B. Cultural
C. Psychological
D. Environmental

405. Invisibility is a communication barrier of:
A. Physiological
B. Cultural
C. Psychological
D. Environmental

406. Levels of knowledge is the communication barrier of:
A. Physiological
B. Cultural
C. Psychological
D. Environmental

407. Valuable items like money, jewellery belonging to patients to be sent to the office of:
A. Administrator
B. Nursing superintendent
C. Resident medical officer
D. Director

408. Neglected mouth care are all *except:*
A. Gingivitis
B. Parotitis
C. Conjunctivitis
D. Glossitis

409. The bandage applied for the head is called:
A. Spical
B. Spiral
C. Circular
D. Capline

---

401 A 402 A 403 A 404 C 405 D 406 B 407 A
408 C 409 D

410. One of the major health problems in India is:
A. Viral hepatitis
B. Tuberculosis
C. Brucellosis
D. Yellow fever

411. One of the Deaconess of the early Christian period:
A. Marcella
B. Paula
C. St. Elizabeth of hungary
D. Phoeba

412. The act of the feeling with the fingers or hands is termed as:
A. Inspection
B. Palpation
C. Percussion
D. Auscultation

413. Anorexia denotes:
A. Loss of sleep
B. Loss of appetite
C. Excess hunger
D. Excess thirst

414. In cardiac pulmonary resuscitation the primary intervention is to:
A. Keep the airway patent
B. Improve the circulation
C. Induce comfort
D. Immobile the patient

415. Gradual return of body temperature:
A. Crisis
B. Lysis
C. Pyrexia
D. None of these

416. Low O_2 content in the blood is called:
A. Anoxia
B. Asphyxia
C. Hypoxia
D. None of these

417. For effective communication:
A. Feed back is essential
B. Sender and receiver is a must
C. Message is very important
D. Proper channel

418. Sharp instruments are sterilized by:
A. Immersing in disinfectants
B. Boiling
C. Flaming
D. Cleaning with soap

---

410 B 411 D 412 B 413 B 414 A 415 B 416 C
417 A 418 A

419. One of the nursing leader:
A. Adelacide mutting
B. Indira Gandhi
C. Febiola
D. Sofia

420. The best health education aid is:
A. Only audio
B. Only visual
C. Combined audio and visual
D. Stimulants all the senses

421. In case of first aid in fracture the following is to be done:
A. Clean and dress the wound
B. Apply a cast
C. Immobilise with a splint
D. Reduce the fracture

422. Darker red colour blood is seen in:
A. Artery bleed
B. Arteriole bleed
C. Capillary bleed
D. Venous bleed

423. Inflammation of the parotid gland is:
A. Glossitis
B. Gingivitis
C. Stomatitis
D. Parotitis

424. In emergency situation maintain:
A. Airway
B. Breathing
C. Circulation
D. All the above

425. Formulating goal and nursing intervention in nursing process is:
A. Planning
B. Implementation
C. Evaluation
D. Assessment

426. To examine the female genitalia and genital tract, the patients should be placed in position:
A. Prone
B. Supine
C. Knee chest
D. Sitting

427. Abnormally elevated heart rate above 100 beats per minute is known as:
A. Tachycardia
B. Bradycardia
C. Dysrhythmia
D. None of these

---

419 C 420 D 421 C 422 D 423 D 424 A 425 A
426 C 427 A

428. **Discontinuity of bone is called:**
A. Fracture
B. Dislocation
C. Sprain
D. Strain

429. **Hand washing is the best way to prevent:**
A. Contamination
B. Cross infection
C. Gravity
D. Infection

430. **The type of bandage used to hold scrotal dressing in position is:**
A. T. bandage
B. Crepe bandage
C. Triangular bandage
D. Capulin bandage

431. **Water is lost from the body through:**
A. Perspiration
B. Expiration
C. Urine and feces
D. All of the above

432. **Sudden return of body temperature to normal:**
A. Crisis
B. Lysis
C. Pyrexia
D. None of these

433. **Administering the medication on the body cavity is known as:**
A. Insufflation
B. Instillation
C. Infusion
D. Inhalation

434. **Stomach wash is otherwise known as:**
A. Lavage
B. Gavage
C. Irrigation
D. None of these

435. **A stiffening of the body after death is:**
A. Rigor mortis
B. Contracture
C. Keloids
D. None of these

436. **The individual's feelings of the security and sense of self esteem develops at the time of:**
A. Adult
B. Older
C. Preschool
D. Birth

---

428 A 429 B 430 A 431 D 432 A 433 B 434 A
435 A 436 A

437. Meaning for p.r.n. in the standing order is:

A. Before meals
B. Start immediately
C. As necessary
D. Once in a day

438. The abdominal binder is used for the following purpose *except:*

A. To retain abdominal dressing
B. To apply pressure
C. Immobilization
D. Support the abdomen

439. Act of urination is known as:

A. Polyuria
B. Pyuria
C. Micturation
D. Anuria

440. 'STAT' dose of medication is administered:

A. Once a day
B. At bed time
C. At once
D. Three times a day

441. The respiratory center is governed by:

A. Hypothalamus
B. Medulla oblongata
C. Cerebral cortex
D. Cerebellum

442. The term universal donor refers to the person with blood group:

A. B
B. A
C. AB
D. O

443. Pulse pressure is:

A. Difference between diastolic and systolic pressure
B. Ratio between systolic and diastolic pressure
C. Addition of systolic and diastolic pressure
D. Division of systolic and diastolic pressure

444. An ideal method of assessing the fluid loss of an edematous patient is:

A. Maintaining intake and output chart
B. Measuring daily weight
C. Measuring girth daily
D. By checking anthropometric measurement

---

437 C 438 C 439 C 440 C 441 B 442 D 443 A
444 A

445. **Passing of more volume of urine than normal is:**
   A. Oliguria
   B. Pyuria
   C. Haematuria
   D. Polyuria

446. **Epistaxis is:**
   A. Vomiting of blood
   B. Coughing up of blood
   C. Bleeding from rectum
   D. Bleeding from nose

447. **The following comfort device is used to relieve dyspnea:**
   A. Bed cradle
   B. Aircushion
   C. Foot board
   D. Back rest

448. **Brown crest formed on the lips teeth due to poor oral hygiene is:**
   A. Calculus
   B. Pyorrhea
   C. Sordes
   D. Parotitis

449. **The term 'ENCODER' refers to:**
   A. Sender
   B. Receiver
   C. Feedback
   D. Message

450. **The term 'Victim' is referred to:**
   A. First aider
   B. Injured person
   C. Witnessed person
   D. Rescuer

451. **A delusion is:**
   A. False belief
   B. False perception
   C. True belief
   D. True perception

452. **Sense of smell is carried by:**
   A. Optic nerve
   B. Auditory nerve
   C. Vestibular nerve
   D. Olfactory nerve

453. **Inability to get sleep is:**
   A. Hyperapnea
   B. Apnea
   C. Insomnia
   D. Anaemia

---

445 D 446 D 447 D 448 C 449 A 450 B 451 A
452 D 453 C

454. Following are the characteristics of pulse *except:*

A. Rate
B. Rhythm
C. Volume
D. Degree

455. The high blood pressure is termed as:

A. Hypotension
B. Hypovolemic shock
C. Hypertension
D. Hypervolemic shock

456. Presence of albumin in the urine is termed as:

A. Oliguria
B. Anuria
C. Albuminuria
D. Dysuria

457. Use of bedside railing is:

A. Considered as safety
B. Therapeutic safety
C. Comfort
D. None of these

458. Specific gravity of the urine is checked with:

A. Lactometer
B. Urinometer
C. Audiometer
D. Barometer

459. The head quarters of TNAI is in:

A. Chennai
B. Kolkata
C. Mumbai
D. New Delhi

460. An act is:

A. A draft
B. A licence
C. A written law
D. Bill

461. Which among the following are some of the common legal hazards or act of negligence in nursing ?

1. Slippery floors
2. Defective electrical equipments
3. Inadequate protection from stray animals
4. Absence of bedside rails for restless patients:

A. 1, 2, 3
B. 2, 3, 4
C. 1, 2, 4
D. 1, 2, 3, 4

---

454 D 455 C 456 C 457 A 458 B 459 D 460 C
461 C

462. **The characteristics of maintaining nurse-patient relationship include all *except:***
   A. Empathy
   B. Genuiness
   C. Trust
   D. Negligence

463. **Which one of the following is the dimension of health?**
   A. Physical
   B. Mental
   C. Social
   D. All the above

464. **A person has got hip bone fracture. The judgement is done by looking at the legs:**
   A. Rotated internally
   B. Held in the flexed position
   C. Moved away from the body's midline
   D. Shorter than the leg of the unaffected area

465. **The signs and symptoms of pressure sore are the following *except:***
   A. Redness
   B. Tenderness
   C. Warmth
   D. Unconsiousness

466. **The solutions used for mouthwash are the following *except:***
   A. $KMnO_4$
   B. H_2O_2
   C. Gentian violet
   D. NaCl

467. **Tridosha theory of disease is of:**
   A. Indian origin
   B. Greek origin
   C. Egyptian origin
   D. Chinese origin

468. **What is the ratio between cardiac massage and artificial respiration while giving CPR?**
   A. 1 : 1
   B. 2 : 2
   C. 10 : 1
   D. 15 : 2

469. **Complications of neglected mouth includes all of the following *except:***
   A. Stomatitis
   B. Gingivitis
   C. Halitosis
   D. Gastritis

470. **Alopacia refers to:**
   A. Loss of skin
   B. Loss of smell
   C. Loss of sweat
   D. Loss of hairs

---

462 D 463 D 464 C 465 D 466 C 467 A 468 C
469 D 470 D

471. The data which is observable and measurable during physical examination is known as:
A. Subjective data
B. Objective data
C. Statistical data
D. Simple data

472. The data which is obtained from patient during physical examination is known as:
A. Subjective data
B. Objective data
C. Statistical data
D. Simple data

473. Diffusion of blood is seen in:
A. Artery bleed
B. Arteriole bleed
C. Capillary bleed
D. Venous bleed

474. Source of secondary data is *except:*
A. Medical record
B. Patient
C. Family members
D. Healthcare team

475. Sitz bath is given to the patient who underwent:
A. Appendicectomy
B. Mastoidectomy
C. Rectal surgery
D. Cataract surgery

476. In heat cramps there will be:
A. Potassium depletion
B. Potassium overload
C. Sodium depletion
D. Sodium overload

477. Neurotoxic poisonous snake is:
A. Pit viper
B. Striped krait
C. Russels viper
D. Rat snake

478. Acetic acid dissolves in:
A. Albumin
B. Phosphate
C. Glucose
D. None of these

479. The term hyperpyrexia is used when the body temperature is above:
A. 105.8 F
B. 104 F
C. 103 F
D. 102 F

480. The amount of air inspired and expired during normal respiration is known as:
A. Vital capacity
B. Tidal volume
C. Residual volume
D. Minute volume

471 B 472 A 473 C 474 B 475 C 476 C 477 A
478 B 479 A 480 B

481. **Most effective method of dystroying micro organism is:**
   A. Dry heat B. Moist heat
   C. Cold sterilization D. Steam under pressure

482. **Haemoptysis due to:**
   A. Bleeding from gum B. Bleeding from lungs
   C. Bleeding from stomach D. Bleeding from nose

483. **Chyne strokes respiration denotes:**
   A. Easy to breath
   B. Long pause of breathing
   C. Absence of breathing
   D. Series of respiration follows deeper and noises

484. **Somnabulism is a:**
   A. Sleep talk B. Dream
   C. Sleep walk D. Nightmare

485. **An instrument used to examine rectum is:**
   A. Sigmoidoscope B. Proctoscope
   C. Autoscope D. Laryngoscope

486. **Sitz bath improves in:**
   A. Circulation B. Nourishment
   C. Healing D. All of these

487. **Drug that inhibit the cough reflex are known as:**
   A. Antiemetic B. Antitussive
   C. Astrigents D. Antipyretics

488. **A patient with pyrexia will be expected to have invariably:**
   A. Dyspnea B. High blood pressure
   C. Tachycardia D. Chest pain

489. **For sterile specimen of urine it should be collected during voiding from:**
   A. First stream B. Mid-stream
   C. Last stream D. Any portion

490. **Acetic acid dissolves:**
   A. Albumin B. Phosphates
   C. Sugar D. All of the above

---

481 D 482 C 483 D 484 C 485 B 486 D 487 B
488 C 489 B 490 B

491. **Artificial feeding is also known as:**
A. Gavage
B. Lavage
C. Suction
D. None of these

492. **Nurse's day is internationally celebrated on:**
A. 5th Sep.
B. 12th May
C. 7th April
D. 1st Dec.

493. **The sites of intramuscular injection are all *except:***
A. Vastus lateralis
B. Abdomen
C. Gluteal region
D. Dettoid

494. **The transfer of heat in the form of waves is called:**
A. Conduction
B. Convection
C. Radiation
D. Evaporation

495. **Position given to a patient while carrying out vaginal examination:**
A. Supine
B. Lithotomy
C. Trendelenburg's
D. Lateral

496. **The most important electrolyte of intracellular fluid is:**
A. Sodium
B. Calcuim
C. Chloride
D. Potassium

497. **A foly catheter operates by the principles of:**
A. Inertia
B. Gravity
C. Diffusion
D. Osmosis

498. **Dyspepsia means difficulty in:**
A. Swallowing
B. Urination
C. Digestion
D. Belching

499. **Hand washing removes the dirt by:**
A. Mechanical method
B. Chemical method
C. Physical method
D. None of these

500. **An oil retention enema is given to:**
A. Protect mucous membrane
B. Check local bleeding
C. Soften faeces
D. Relieve local irritation

---

491 A 492 B 493 B 494 C 495 B 496 D 497 B
498 A 499 A 500 C

501. An example for isotonic solution is:
A. 0.45% Sodium Chloride NaCl
B. 3% NaCl
C. 0.9% NaCl
D. 5% NaCl

502. Movement of fluid from higher concentration to lower concentration is:
A. Osmosis
B. Osmolality
C. Filtration
D. Diffusion

503. A person supports the microbes providing living condition is:
A. Host
B. Agent
C. Case
D. Individual

504. Fluid volume deficit is manifested by:
A. Increased thirst
B. Giddiness
C. High BP
D. High Fever

505. Fall of blood pressure in upright position is called:
A. Syncope
B. Dizziness
C. Hypotension
D. Orthostatic hypotension

506. The area of auscultation from third intercoastal space to left atrium is:
A. Erbs Point
B. Tricuspid area
C. Apical area
D. Pulmonic area

507. Tinea pedis (athletes foot) is:
A. Bacterial infection
B. Fungal infection
C. Viral infection
D. Allergic infection

508. Excision of body part is termed:
A. Tomy
B. Ectomy
C. Scopy
D. Plasty

509. Protrusion of an organ through a loose sac is called:
A. Hernia
B. Perforation
C. Inversion
D. Retraction

---

501 C 502 A 503 A 504 A 505 D 506 D 507 B
508 B 509 A

510. Paralysis of both arms and legs is:

A. Hemiplegia
B. Paraplegia
C. Quadriplegia
D. Tetraplegia

511. Common health problems in old age are the following, except:

A. Incontinence
B. Hearing loss
C. Insomnia
D. Gastric ulcer

512. Distance followed while checking visual acuity is:

A. 6 feet
B. 20 feet
C. 16 feet
D. 11 feet

513. Communication process is initiated by a:

A. Stimulus
B. Person
C. Environment
D. Channel

514. An example for auditory medium of communication is:

A. Touch
B. Sight
C. Observation
D. Spoken word

515. An example for sensory medium of communication is:

A. Touch
B. Sight
C. Observation
D. Spoken word

516. An example for visual medium of communication is:

A. Sight
B. Taste
C. Observation
D. Spoken word

517. The other name for fever is:

A. Pyrexia
B. Pyorrhoea
C. Palpitation
D. Pyrogen

518. The instrument used for auscultation is:

A. Otoscope
B. Auroscope
C. Stethoscope
D. Bronchoscope

519. The instrument used to examine the ears is:

A. Auroscope
B. Otoscope
C. Bronchoscope
D. All of them

---

510 C 511 D 512 B 513 A 514 D 515 A 516 A
517 A 518 C 519 A

520. Hardened fecal content results in:

A. Constipation
B. Diarrhea
C. Obstipation
D. Steatorrhea

521. The amount of blood pumped per minute is:

A. Cardiac output
B. Pulse pressure
C. Blood pressure
D. Cardiac pressure

522. The difference between the apical and radial pulse rate is:

A. Pulse deficit
B. Heart rate
C. Pulse amplitude
D. Dysrhythmia

523. A procedure that facilitates bowel elimination is:

A. Lavage
B. Gavage
C. Enema
D. Diversion

524. An equipment used to measure oxygen (O2) saturation is:

A. Apparatus
B. Catheter
C. Oxmetry
D. Doisimeter

525. A position in which the head end is elevated and the body is upright:

A. Lateral
B. Prone
C. Supine
D. Fowler's

526. Sodium is a:

A. Fluid
B. Acid
C. Base
D. Electrolyte

527. Regulation of fluid and electrolytes are maintained by:

A. Brain
B. Lungs
C. Kidney
D. Heart

528. Preparation of patient for surgery is done during:

A. Preoperative phase
B. Postoperative phase
C. Intraoperative phase
D. Admission phase

529. The standard safety precautions followed all over the world is:

A. National precaution
B. Global precaution
C. Universal precaution
D. State precaution

---

520 A 521 A 522 A 523 C 524 C 525 D 526 D
527 C 528 A 529 C

530. The hospital acquired infection is otherwise known:
A. Bacterial infection
B. Auto infection
C. Cross infection
D. Nosocomial infection

531. Infection by one's own self is:
A. Bacterial infection
B. Auto infection
C. Cross infection
D. Nosocomial infection

532. The causative factor of stress is:
A. Stressor
B. Stimulation
C. Adoptor
D. Acceptor

533. One of the hazard, associated with immobility is:
A. Foot drop
B. Palpitation
C. Regurgitation
D. None of these

534. Visual examination of the body is:
A. Inspection
B. Palpation
C. Auscultation
D. Manipulation

535. Examination of the body by using hand is:
A. Inspection
B. Palpation
C. Auscultation
D. Manipulation

536. The heat is lost from the body through:
A. Skin, lungs, and kidney
B. Skin, lungs, kidney and heart
C. Skin, lungs, kidney and brain
D. Skin, lungs, kidney and liver

537. The heat is lost from the body through all of the following, except:
A. Skin
B. Lungs
C. Kidney
D. Liver

538. Respiration that gradually become deeper and noisy is:
A. Stridor
B. Apnea
C. Dyspnea
D. Capnea

539. Lack of oxygen to the tissues can be identified by:
A. Cyanosis
B. Halitosis
C. Sprirosis
D. Heptosis

---

530 D 531 B 532 A 533 A 534 A 535 B 536 A
537 D 538 A 539 A

540. One of the major guidelines for nursing practice is:
A. Philosophy
B. Process recording
C. Nursing process
D. Nurses report

541. Hierarchy of basic human needs was developed by:
A. Maslow
B. Duffer
C. Florence
D. Amelia

542. The word that may be used to describe a concept is:
A. Science
B. Idea
C. Fact
D. Truth

543. About 21 problems of a patient was listed by:
A. Florence
B. Henderson
C. Abdulla
D. Maslow

544. The data collected through by seeing, hearing and feeling is:
A. Subjective
B. Objective
C. Both of them
D. None of these

545. Foot care is necessary for patient, who are:
A. Mobile
B. Ambulant
C. Bedridden
D. Mobile with assistance

546. The type of bed prepared by allowing the patient to sit on the chair is:
A. Open bed
B. Closed bed
C. Surgical bed
D. Occupied bed

547. A method of evaluating nursing care through patient records is:
A. Nursing review
B. Nursing process
C. Nursing audit
D. Nursing evaluation

548. The stages of grieving and death was given by:
A. Orlando
B. Sr Nancy
C. Dugas
D. Ross

549. Following pneumonectomy surgery, the nurse should turn the patient to:
A. Operated side
B. Unoperated side
C. Both
D. None

540 C 541 A 542 B 543 B 544 B 545 C 546 D
547 C 548 D 549 A

550. Deep vein thrombosis can be prevented by:
A. Leg exercise
B. Breathing exercise
C. Abdominal exercise
D. All of these

551. The transfer order of a patient will be written by:
A. Nurse
B. Doctor
C. Head nurse
D. Tutor

552. Allowing a patient to stay in the hospital for observation, investigation and treatment is:
A. Admission
B. Discharge
C. Transfer in
D. Transfer out

553. Recurrent altered state of consciousness that occurs for sustained period restoring energy and well-being is:
A. Comfort
B. Sleep
C. Rest
D. Activity

554. The procedures used to keep objects on a sterile are completely free from all microbes is:
A. Medical asepsis
B. Surgical asepsis
C. Barrier technique
D. Reverse barrier technique

555. The method of introducing large quantity of medicines on fluids is called:
A. Infusion
B. Transfusion
C. Injection
D. Inoculation

556. The rule or principle that governs right conduct is called:
A. Communication
B. Profession
C. Ethics
D. Standards

557. Facial expression is, which form of communication:
A. Verbal
B. Non-verbal
C. Meta
D. Grapevine

558. A silvery liquid metal used in the thermometer is:
A. Mercury
B. Lead
C. Iron
D. Copper

---

550 A 551 B 552 A 553 B 554 B 555 A 556 C
557. B 558. A

559. **Short wave diathermy is an example of local application of:**
A. Dry heat
B. Moist heat
C. Dry cold
D. Moist cold

560. **The fourteen human needs are explained by the nursing theorist:**
A. Abdulla
B. Henderson
C. Watson
D. Orem

561. **The body temperature is lowest, when it is taken by:**
A. Mouth
B. Axilla
C. Rectum
D. Ear canal

562. **The commonest route of administration of insulin is:**
A. Intradermal
B. Intravenous
C. Intramural
D. Subcutaneous

563. **The device used to visualize the bronchus is:**
A. Laryngoscope
B. Bronchoscope
C. Otoscope
D. Gastroscopy

564. **The device used to see the stomach is:**
A. Gastroscope
B. Laryngoscope
C. Foetoscope
D. Colonoscope

565. **The device used to examine the colon is:**
A. Colonoscope
B. Laryngoscope
C. Stethoscope
D. Gastroscopy

566. **Lumbar puncture is done to withdraw:**
A. Lymph
B. Cerebro spinal fluid (CSF)
C. Blood
D. Pleural fluid

567. **Thoracocentesis is done to withdraw:**
A. Lymph
B. CSF
C. Pleural fluid
D. Pericardial fluid

568. **Excessive contact with cold causes:**
A. Frost bite
B. Scald
C. Burns
D. Heat stroke

569. **The level of most basic needs of human needs is:**
A. Physiologic
B. Safety and security
C. Love and belonging
D. Self-actualization

---

559 A 560 B 561 B 562 D 563 B 564 A 565 A
566 B 567 C 568 A 569 A

570. Of all the physiologic needs, the most essential one is:
A. Food B. Water
C. Climatic D. Oxygen

571. Handwashing and sterile technique includes in which level of human needs?
A. Physiologic
B. Safety and security
C. Self-esteem
D. Love and belonging

572. Individuals learn health beliefs and values at:
A. Family B. School
C. Peers D. Friends

573. One element of healthy community is:
A. Meeting all the needs
B. Offering access to healthcare services
C. Has mixed groups
D. Concerned with air and water.

574. The largest subculture group of the healthcare system is:
A. Nurses B. Physicians
C. Social workers D. Physiotherapist

575. The one defined as a disease is:
A. Fluid overload B. Hypoxia
C. Rheumatoid arthritis D. Hyperpyrexia

576. Among the four concepts to nursing theories, the most important concept is:
A. Person B. Environment
C. Health D. Nursing

577. The one does not pertaining to care in a hospital is:
A. Acute care provider B. Inpatient
C. Outpatient D. Flight nursing

578. How often a nurse document progress notes?
A. End of the day B. Before caring
C. During caring D. After caring

570 D 571 B 572 A 573 B 574 A 575 C 576 A
577 D 578 C

579. Patient's complains about nausea, is an example for:
A. Subjective data
B. Objective data
C. Signs, symptoms
D. Overt data

580. Altered health maintenance is an example of:
A. Collaborative problem
B. Interdisciplinary
C. Medical problem
D. Nursing problem

581. The form, a nurse should refer to know the trends in a patient's vital signs is:
A. Admission record
B. Activity flow chart
C. Nurses report
D. Graphic chart

582. Infections in the neonate are less likely to mothers, who provide nutrition, through:
A. Breast milk
B. Water
C. Formula feed
D. Cow's milk

583. Bonding occurs at:
A. 6 months
B. 3 weeks
C. Soon after birth
D. 12 months

584. The ability to reproduce in the adolescent is defined as:
A. Maturation
B. Adulthood
C. Puberty
D. Latency

585. The leading cause of death in adolescent is:
A. Accidents
B. Substance abuse
C. Sexually transmitted diseases
D. Unhealthy diets

586. In the nursing diagnosis, a nurse will make for a patient, who says he lives alone is:
A. Social isolation
B. Powerlessness
C. Risk for injury
D. Risk for falls

587. A nurse using the communication technique of silence to assists the family of:
A. Communicate with the patient
B. Plan for discharge
C. Organize their thoughts
D. Decrease anxiety

579 A 580 D 581 D 582 A 583 C 584 C 585 A
586 A 587 C

588. Nurses play a vital role in patient teaching because of their:
A. Need for self actualization
B. Expertise in health care
C. Desire to help others
D. Ability to provide health care

589. In recording BP of 120/80 mm Hg, the 120 represents the:
A. Pulse rate B. Systolic pressure
C. Diastolic pressure D. Pulse deficit

590. An equipment, necessary to assess the apical pulse is:
A. Sphygmomanometer
B. Clinical thermometer
C. Stethoscope
D. Doppler apparatus

591. With aging, BP is often higher due to:
A. Loss of muscle tone
B. Changes in diet
C. Decreased peripheral resistance
D. Decreased elasticity in arterial walls.

592. Palpation is a physical assessment technique that uses the sense of:
A. Intuition B. Vision
C. Hearing D. Touch

593. The bell of the stethoscope is used to hear:
A. Bowel sounds B. Lung sounds
C. Heart sounds D. Tympanic sounds

594. The one does not used for assessing orientation in mental status examination is:
A. Time B. Place
C. Person D. Consciousness

595. The smallest infectious agents capable of causing an infection are:
A. Bacteria B. Virus
C. Moulds D. Yeasts

588 B 589 B 590 C 591 D 592 D 593 C 594 D
595 B

596. **Complementary and alternative therapies are:**
   A. Safe interventions
   B. Used by a minority of patients
   C. Relatively new
   D. Recognized by Indian Nursing Council (INC)

597. **A combination of traditional medical care and complementary alternative therapy is called:**
   A. Integrative care
   B. Holism
   C. Allopath
   D. Chinese medicine

598. **An abnormal, unexpected response to a drug is:**
   A. Drug intolerance
   B. Cumulative effect
   C. Idiosyncratic effect
   D. Anaphylactic reaction

599. **In medication error, the first response by the nurse is:**
   A. Record the error on the medication sheet
   B. Notify the physician
   C. Check the patient's condition
   D. Complete an incident report

600. **Administering therapeutic agents including food outside the alimentary tract is called:**
   A. Parental therapy
   B. External therapy
   C. Nutritional therapy
   D. Intravenous therapy

601. **Drugs or fluids into the bone marrow is called:**
   A. Intraperitoneal injection
   B. Intrathecal injection
   C. Intraosteous injection
   D. Infusion

602. **The nerve, which may get injured during faulty in injection technique is:**
   A. Optic nerve
   B. Olfactory nerve
   C. Sciatica nerve
   D. Radial nerve

603. **Euthanasia means:**
   A. Mercy killing
   B. Murder
   C. Suicide
   D. Delayed death

---

596 B 597 A 598 C 599 C 600 A 601 C 602 C
603 A

604. **The stages of death is described by:**
A. Sr Nancy B. Dugar
C. Kubler Ross D. Florence

605. **An example of inhalation type of anesthetic drug is:**
A. Diazepam B. Morphine
C. Halothane D. Midazolam

606. **The person, who described just nursing as a process is:**
A. Orlando B. Lydia Hal
C. Widenback D. Park

607. **Patients perceptions about their health problems are grouped as:**
A. Objective data B. Overt data
C. Subjective data D. Personal data

608. **Paint or varnish stain on linen is best removed by:**
A. Kerosene B. Spirit
C. Turpentine D. Petrol

609. **Discharge summary of the patient to be written by:**
A. Ward nurse B. Head nurse
C. Doctor D. Tutor

610. **The urine that remains in the bladder is:**
A. Residual urine B. Contaminated urine
C. Total urine D. Cloudy urine

611. **The residual urine is one that remains in the bladder:**
A. Before voiding B. After voiding
C. During voiding D. Always

612. **An organized conversation with a patient to obtain health history is:**
A. Physical examination B. Interview
C. Health education D. Assessment

613. **The purpose of record keeping is:**
A. Follow-up B. Education
C. Research D. All of these

---

604 C 605 D 606 B 607 C 608 D 609 C 610 A
611 D 612 B 613 D

614. **Health belief model was developed by:**
   A. Florence B. Rosenstach
   C. Virginia D. Preplan

615. **Roy has developed _______________ model:**
   A. Self-care B. In logic needs
   C. Adaptation D. Health belief

616. **The process of sanitizing and preserving human body is:**
   A. Embalming B. Disinfecting
   C. Branding D. Preserving

617. **Forensic autopsy is used to determine the cause of:**
   A. Death B. Disease
   C. Result of treatment D. None of these

618. **Stat means:**
   A. Hour B. When needed
   C. At once D. Any time

619. **Urine for Heys test is to detect:**
   A. Protein B. Albumin
   C. Bile salt D. Bile pigment

620. **For blood transfusion the size of the IV cannula to be used is:**
   A. 18G B. 22G
   C. 21G D. 26G

621. **Contraindication for nasogastric feeding is:**
   A. Gastric surgery B. Paralytic ileus
   C. Gastric bleeding D. All of above

622. **Indication for chest drainage is:**
   A. Tibial fracture B. Pneumothorax
   C. Abdominal trauma D. Cardiac failure

623. **Callus is caused by:**
   A. Friction B. Injury
   C. Infection D. None of these

---

614 B 615 C 616 A 617 C 618 C 619 C 620 A
621 D 622 B 623 A

624. Hazard of restraints is:

A. Nerve damage
B. Pressure sore
C. Foot drop
D. All of above

625. Example of medical diagnosis is:

A. Pain
B. Fatigue
C. Edema
D. Hypertension

624 D 625 D

CHAPTER 2

Community Health Nursing

1. **A disease that is interpreted as being punishment for one's past sins in some cultures is:**
   A. Leprosy
   B. Tuberculosis
   C. HIV
   D. Syphilis

2. **In ancient India, the celebrated authorities in Ayurvedic medicine were *except:***
   A. Atreya
   B. Charaka
   C. Susruta
   D. Hippocrates

3. **Barefoot doctor and acupuncture is the system of:**
   A. India
   B. China
   C. Egypt
   D. Greek

4. **One applied to non-living things and physical factors with which man is in constant interaction is the:**
   A. Physical environment
   B. Biological environment
   C. Macro environment
   D. Micro environment

5. **The study of man as a social being in his total environment is the:**
   A. Social medicine
   B. Indian medicine
   C. Preventive medicine
   D. None of these

6. **The time interval between invasion by an infections agent and appearance of the just sign / symptom of the disease in question is the:**
   A. Latent period
   B. Quarantine
   C. Incubation period
   D. Terminal period

---

1 A　2 B　3 B　4 A　5 A　6 C

7. **The subjective component of well being is referred to as:**
   A. Standard of living
   B. Quality of work
   C. Quality of life
   D. Physical quality of life

8. **The following are the components of level of living *except:***
   A. Health
   B. Environment
   C. Education
   D. Occupation

9. **The process of continuous progressive improvement of the health status of a population is:**
   A. Community development
   B. Block development
   C. Society development
   D. Health development

10. **The floating tip of the ice berg represents:**
    A. Clinical cases
    B. Apparent cases
    C. Latent cases
    D. Undiagnosed cases

11. **Sleeping sickness is transmitted by:**
    A. Black fly
    B. Tsetse fly
    C. Sand fly
    D. House fly

12. **Screening of immigrants for infectious disease is:**
    A. Mass screening
    B. Selective screening
    C. Prospective screening
    D. Prescriptive screening

13. **80% of the cholera cases can be diagnosed within a few minute by:**
    A. Culture exam
    B. Biochemical exam
    C. Microscopical exam
    D. None of these

14. **Immunity comes from the bone-marrow derived lymphocytes is:**
    A. Humoral
    B. Cellular
    C. Passive
    D. Herd

---

7 C 8 B 9 D 10 A 11 B 12 C 13 C
14 A

15. **The part in under five clinic's symbol that represents mother's felt need is:**
    A. Base B. Centre
    C. Sides D. Apex

16. **Cohort study is also known as *except:***
    A. Prospective study B. Retrospective study
    C. Forward looking study D. Incidence study

17. **An infection that always occur in association with hepatitis B is:**
    A. Hepatitis A B. Hepatitis E
    C. Hepatitis D D. Hepatitis C

18. **The central family planning institute was established in:**
    A. Chennai B. Mumbai
    C. Kolkata D. New Delhi

19. **The recommended land size for higher elementary schools by the school health committee is:**
    A. 1.5 acres B. 10 acres
    C. 15 acres D. 20 acres

20. **The major antibody responsible for immediate allergic anaphylactic reaction is:**
    A. IgE B. IgG
    C. IgM D. IgA

21. **Progeny of primitive man is:**
    A. Traditional healer
    B. Magician
    C. Religious man
    D. None of these

22. **Father of Indian surgery is:**
    A. Susruta B. Charaka
    C. Atreya D. Vaghbhata

23. **An epidemiologist who studied the epidemiology of cholera:**
    A. John Simon B. William Budd
    C. Johnsnow D. James Lind

---

15 D 16 B 17 C 18 D 19 B 20 B 21 A
22 A 23 C

24. **International conference at Alma-Ata held in the year:**
    A. 1970 B. 1972
    C. 1974 D. 1978

25. **Health means absence of disease is the concept of:**
    A. Ecology B. Holistic
    C. Biomedical D. Psychosocial

26. **Infant mortality, life expectancy at age one and literacy are the consolidated index of:**
    A. Quality of life B. Physical quality of life
    C. Standard of living D. Child health

27. **In the late 19th century the multiple cause theory was overshadowed by:**
    A. Germ theory B. Holistic theory
    C. Biomedical theory D. None of these

28. **Submerged portion of ice-berg represents:**
    A. Carrier B. Clinical case
    C. Undiagnosed case D. Latent case

29. **Tear out by roots is the literal meaning of:**
    A. Isolation B. Elimination
    C. Eradication D. Transmission

30. **On going measurement of performance of a health service refers to:**
    A. Evaluation B. Surveillance
    C. Scrutinization D. Monitoring

31. **Population strategy is the approach recommended by WHO for:**
    A. Primary prevention
    B. Secondary prevention
    C. Tertiary prevention
    D. Primordial prevention

32. **The process of enabling people to improve health is:**
    A. Health education B. Health promotion
    C. Rehabilitation D. Specific protection

---

24 D 25 C 26 B 27 A 28 C 29 C 30 B
31 D 32 B

33. **Any restriction to perform an activity is termed as:**
A. Dysuse
B. Handicap
C. Disability
D. Impairment

34. **The pattern of disease in a community described in terms of:**
A. Community participation
B. Community evaluation
C. Community treatment
D. Community diagnosis

35. **The study of defined population is a unit of:**
A. Epidemiology
B. Clinical medicine
C. Social medicine
D. Anthropology

36. **The ratio of the incidence of the disease or death among exposed and the incidence among non-exposed is:**
A. Attributable risk
B. Relative risk
C. Population at risk
D. High risk

37. **Selective partial limitation of freedom of movement is:**
A. Absolute quarantine
B. Isolation
C. Modified quarantine
D. Segregation

38. **The science of the health of travelers is:**
A. Entomology
B. Epidemiology
C. Ecology
D. Emporiatrics

39. **Presumptive identification of unrecognized disease is:**
A. Mass screening
B. Selective screening
C. Prospective screening
D. Prescriptive screening

40. **India was declared smallpox free in the year:**
A. 1977
B. 1975
C. 1973
D. 1971

41. **In India people talk of curing snake bites by:**
A. Mantras
B. Traditional healer
C. Priest
D. Magic

42. **The science of Ayurveda gradually developed from the medical knowledge in the:**
A. Rig Veda
B. Yajur Veda
C. Sama Veda
D. Atharva Veda

---

33 C 34 D 35 A 36 A 37 C 38 D 39 D
40 A 41 A 42 D

43. **Public health was born in:**
    A. Greek B. Egypt
    C. Rome D. China

44. **The first case of a communicable disease introduced into the population unit being studied is the:**
    A. Primary case B. Secondary case
    C. Index case D. Risk case

45. **The level of noise, a normal conversation produces:**
    A. 20 to 30 dB B. 40 to 50 dB
    C. 50 to 60 dB D. 60 to 70 dB

46. **The stage in which there is high birth and death rate:**
    A. Early expanding B. High stationary
    C. Declining D. Low stationary

47. **Lung function test is an example for:**
    A. Mass screening B. High risk screening
    C. Multiphasic screening D. Selective screening

48. **An animal associated with laptospirosis is:**
    A. Dog B. Cat
    C. Rat D. Pig

49. **Purification of water can be done in the home easily by:**
    A. Boiling B. Filteration
    C. Mixing alum D. Adding chlorine

50. **Health survey and planning committee is popularly known as the:**
    A. Bhore committee B. Chadah committee
    C. Mudaliar committee D. Mukerji committee

51. **National health policy was evolved by the govt. of India in the year:**
    A. 1980 B. 1981
    C. 1982 D. 1983

52. **Retarded intrauterine foetal growth results in:**
    A. Low birth weight babies B. Small far date babies
    C. Pre-term babies D. Term babies

---

43 C 44 A 45 A 46 B 47 D 48 C 49 A
50 C 51 D 52 A

53. **The ratio of the incidence of the disease among exposed and non-exposed and the incidence among non-exposed is:**
   A. Attributable risk
   B. High risk
   C. Relative risk
   D. Risk difference

54. **The census is taken in most countries of the world at regular intervals usually of:**
   A. 10 years
   B. 15 years
   C. 5 years
   D. 20 years

55. **The commonly occurring value in a distribution of data is:**
   A. Mean
   B. Median
   C. Range
   D. Mode

56. **Historically in 1747, one who performed a human experiment of soldiers:**
   A. James Lind
   B. Edward Jenner
   C. Finley
   D. John Snow

57. **The one indicator included in WHO list for monitoring progress towards health for all is:**
   A. Health policy indictor
   B. Crude death rate indicator
   C. Literacy rate
   D. Annual growth rate indicator

58. **The requirement indicator of iron intake for lactating mother per day is:**
   A. 32 mg
   B. 35 mg
   C. 40 mg
   D. 45 mg

59. **The amount of breast milk a poor Indian women secret per day during first year is:**
   A. 300 to 400 ml
   B. 400 to 600 ml
   C. 350 to 400 ml
   D. 500 to 600 ml

60. **The apgar scare of 4 to 6 indicates:**
   A. Moderate depression
   B. Prompt action
   C. Severe depression
   D. Death during neonatal period

---

53 C 54 A 55 B 56 A 57 A 58 A 59 B
60 A

61. **The state that has MMR higher than the national average is:**
   A. Andhra Pradesh
   B. Madhya Pradesh
   C. Uttar Pradesh
   D. Rajasthan

62. **The term to be used to include all bio-chemical, structural and functional disorders present at birth is:**
   A. Congenital malformation
   B. Birth defects
   C. Congenital anomaly
   D. All of the above

63. **First time medical examination of school children was carried out in India in the year:**
   A. 1909
   B. 1907
   C. 1908
   D. 1910

64. **The method that kills vibrio cholerae within 30 minutes is:**
   A. Freezing
   B. Boiling
   C. Drying
   D. None of the above

65. **The ability of an infection's agent invade and multiply in a host is:**
   A. Pathogenicity
   B. Prepathogenicity
   C. Infectivity
   D. Virulence

66. **The epidemiological terminology, soil refers to:**
   A. Human host
   B. Disease agent
   C. Environment
   D. Social status

67. **An attribute that is significantly associated with the development of a disease is:**
   A. Agent factor
   B. Host factor
   C. Environmental factor
   D. Risk factor

68. **One way of measuring virulence of an infection's agent is by:**
   A. Attack rate
   B. Incidence rate
   C. Case fatality rate
   D. Morbidity rate

---

61 B 62 D 63 A 64 C 65 A 66 A 67 B
68 A

69. **Case control study is also known, *except:***
   A. Prospective study
   B. Retrospective study
   C. Forward-looking study
   D. Incidence study

70. **Usual or expected frequency of the disease within a geographic area refers to:**
   A. Epidemic
   B. Endemic
   C. Sporadic
   D. Pandemic

71. **The term refers to the first case to come to the attention of the investigator:**
   A. Index case
   B. Primary case
   C. Secondary case
   D. Clinical case

72. **Vaccine that must be stored in the freezer compartment is:**
   A. DPT
   B. BCG
   C. Measles
   D. Typhoid

73. **Immunity of a community or a group of people:**
   A. Active
   B. Passive
   C. Herd
   D. None of these

74. **The immunoglobulin that is transported across the placenta is:**
   A. IgM
   B. IgG
   C. IgA
   D. IgE

75. **Hand washing is an example for ___ disinfection:**
   A. Concurrent
   B. Terminal
   C. Precurrent
   D. Current

76. **Screening of a whole population or a sub-group is the:**
   A. Prospective screening
   B. Prescriptive screening
   C. Mass screening
   D. Selective screening

77. **In India the recent census is taken in the year:**
   A. 2000
   B. 1990
   C. 1980
   D. 1970

---

69 B 70 A 71 C 72 C 73 C 74 B 75 A
76 C 77 A

78. **Per capita space for students in a classroom should be:**
A. 5 sq. ft
B. 15 sq. ft
C. 10 sq. ft
D. 20 sq. ft

79. **Minister for Health and Family Welfare of Govt. of India at present is:**
A. Dr. Thackur
B. Mr. Shatrugan Sinha
C. Dr. Anbumani
D. Miss Mayavathy

80. **Schick test is done to identify the immunity status against:**
A. Diphtheria
B. Measles
C. Mumps
D. German measles

81. **A nationwide family planning programme was launched in India in:**
A. 1952
B. 1950
C. 1955
D. 1953

82. **Great sanitary awakening took place in:**
A. London
B. England
C. Europe
D. America

83. **The concept that viewed the disease due to disequilibrium between man and the environment:**
A. Biomedical
B. Psychosocial
C. Ecological
D. Holistic

84. **The index that is used to know the expectation of life free of disability:**
A. Health index
B. Physical quality of life index
C. Sullivan's index
D. All of these

85. **Sentinal surveillance is used to identify:**
A. Missing cases
B. Clinical cases
C. Undiagnosed cases
D. Latent cases

---

78 C 79 C 80 A 81 A 82 B 83 C 84 C
85 A

86. **Softening of water is recommended when the hardness exceeds __ mg per litre:**
A. 500
B. 450
C. 400
D. 300

87. **The level of noise, people can tolerate without damage to hearing by daily exposure:**
A. Upto 100 dB
B. Upto 85 dB
C. Upto 90 dB
D. Upto 120 dB

88. **An instrument that measures humidity:**
A. Anemometer
B. Barometer
C. Hygrometer
D. Cyclometer

89. **Kala azar is transmitted by:**
A. Tsetse fly
B. Sand fly
C. House fly
D. Black fly

90. **The disease which may be transmitted by eating unwholesome meat:**
A. Amoebiasis
B. Ascariasis
C. Dracunculiasis
D. Taeniasis

91. **The mosquito that lays eggs singly:**
A. Anopheles
B. Culex
C. Aedes
D. Mansonia

92. **The stage in which there is high birth rate and declining death rate:**
A. High stationary
B. Low stationary
C. Late expanding
D. Early expanding

93. **New revised population policy was in the year:**
A. 1976
B. 1986
C. 1966
D. 1956

94. **The lynchpins of the family planning delivery system in India in the village:**
A. Social worker
B. Anganwadi worker
C. Village health nurse
D. Traditional birth attendant

---

86 D 87 B 88 C 89 B 90 A 91 A 92 D
93 B 94 D

95. **In the year 1972, Govt. of India introduced:**
   A. National family welfare programme
   B. All India hospital postpartum programme
   C. Medical termination of pregnancy
   D. National population policy

96. **The headquarters of South East Asia region of W.H.O. is in:**
   A. Dhaka
   B. New Delhi
   C. Thailand
   D. Ceylon

97. **B lymphoid cells are responsible for:**
   A. Cellular immunity
   B. Passive immunity
   C. Humoral immunity
   D. Hard immunity

98. **A test that identifies the person's immune status to diphtheria:**
   A. Lepromin
   B. Tuberculin
   C. Skin clip
   D. Schick

99. **Health survey and development committee was appointed by the Govt. of India in the year:**
   A. 1943
   B. 1942
   C. 1941
   D. 1940

100. **Rh anti D immunoglobulin should be given at ____ weeks of gestation:**
   A. 24
   B. 26
   C. 28
   D. 30

101. **Guthrie test is done to find out the disorders of:**
   A. Carbohydrate metabolism
   B. Amino acid metabolism
   C. Fat metabolism
   D. All the above

102. **The energy value of human milk per 100 ml is:**
   A. 60 Kcal
   B. 70 Kcal
   C. 80 Kcal
   D. 90 Kcal

---

95 C 96 B 97 A 98 D 99 A 100 C 101 A
102 B

103. The principal health worker in ICDS project is the:
A. Balwadi worker
B. Project worker
C. Health guide
D. Anganwadi worker

104. The term that confirms the structural defects at birth as per WHO document is:
A. Congenital malformation
B. Congenital anomaly
C. Birth defects
D. All the above

105. First time medical examination of school children was carried out in:
A. Lucknow
B. Delhi
C. Bombay
D. Baroda

106. The recommended land size for primary school by the school health committee is:
A. 5 acres
B. 10 acres
C. 15 acres
D. 20 acres

107. The ability of an infectious agent to induce clinically apparent illness is:
A. Pathogenicity
B. Infectivity
C. Virulence
D. Prepathogenicity

108. In epidemiological terminology, seed refers to:
A. Human host
B. Environment
C. Culture
D. Disease agent

109. Prevention of the development of risk factors in population is:
A. Primary prevention
B. Primodial prevention
C. Secondary prevention
D. Tertiary prevention

---

103 D 104 B 105 D 106 A 107 A 108 D 109 B

110. Case control studies are often called as:
A. Retrospective study
B. Observational study
C. Incidence study
D. Prospective study

111. The incidence of the disease in the total population minus the incidence of the disease among those who were not exposed is the:
A. Relative risk
B. High risk
C. Population attributable risk
D. Population risk

112. Constant presence of a disease within a given geographic area is:
A. Epidemic
B. Endemic
C. Pandemic
D. Sporadic

113. An inanimate or article capable of transferring disease agent is:
A. Food
B. Faeces
C. Fingers
D. Fomites

114. A diluent to be used for reconstituting the BCG vaccine is:
A. Distilled water
B. Glucose water
C. Saline water
D. Normal saline

115. Primary resistance shown by the bacteria against TB drugs in patient who has:
A. Not received the drug
B. Received the drug
C. Discontinued the drug
D. None of these

116. An infection that is essential a water borne disease is:
A. Hepatitis A
B. Hepatitis E
C. Hepatitis D
D. Hepatitis B

---

110 A 111 C 112 B 113 D 114 D 115 A 116 A

117. The result of the Mantoux test is read after:

A. 24 hours B. 72 hours
C. 48 hours D. 12 hours

118. Koplick's spot is seen in the case of:

A. Measles B. Mumps
C. Diphtheria D. Pertussis

119. Dracunculiasis is a vector borne disease of ____ parasite:

A. Hook worm B. Round worm
C. Guinea worm D. Pin worm

120. Tridosha theory of disease is the significance in:

A. Ayurveda B. Unani
C. Siddha D. Homeopathy

121. Father of public health is:

A. Plague B. Cholera
C. Malaria D. Leprosy

122. Code of personal hygiene was the law of:

A. Manu B. Charaka Samhita
C. Susruta Samhita D. Code of ethics

123. A naval surgeon advocated the intake of fresh fruits and vegetables for the prevention of scurvy:

A. John Snow B. William Budd
C. John Simon D. James Lind

124. Disease is the maladjustment between an organism and the environment is the concept of:

A. Holistic B. Biomedical
C. Ecology D. Psychosocial

125. In immunization against chlorea immunity develops after:

A. 6 days B. 10 days
C. 15 days D. 20 days

126. The components of health system are *except:*

A. Concepts B. Ideas
C. Objects D. Policy

---

117 D 118 A 119 C 120 A 121 B 122 A 123 D
124 C 125 A 126 D

127. **The science of mutual relationship between living organism and their environment is:**
A. Ecology
B. Embriology
C. Etiology
D. Economics

128. **The continuous scrutiny of the factors that determine the occurrence and distribution of disease is the:**
A. Evaluation
B. Surveillance
C. Monitoring
D. Elimination

129. **Imperfect tool in the control of transmission of disease is:**
A. Primary prevention
B. Tertiary prevention
C. Secondary prevention
D. None of these

130. **A disadvantage for a given individual that limits normal role is:**
A. Handicap
B. Impairment
C. Disability
D. Dysuse

131. **The study of cases is a unit of:**
A. Epidemiology
B. Clinical medicine
C. Social medicine
D. Community medicine

132. **The term applied to all those to whom an event could have happened whether it did or not is:**
A. Person at risk
B. Exposed to risk
C. Population at risk
D. High risk

133. **The epidemic usually shows a gradual rise and tails off over a much longer period of time is:**
A. Point source epidemic
B. Modern epidemic
C. Epidemic curve
D. Propagated epidemic

134. **The separation for special consideration, control of observation of some part of a group of persons from others is defined as:**
A. Absolute quarantine
B. Segregation
C. Isolation
D. Quarantine

---

127 A 128 B 129 C 130 A 131 A 132 B 133 D
134 D

135. The period between diagnosis by early detection and diagnosis by other means is:
A. Screening time
B. Time lag
C. Lead time
D. Diagnostic time

136. The requirement of calcium intake for lactating mother per day:
A. 500 mg
B. 1000 mg
C. 1500 mg
D. 1250 mg

137. The first great Indian physician and teacher in Ayurvedic medicine:
A. Charaka
B. Atreya
C. Susruta
D. Vaghbhata

138. The concept that has the basis of the germ theory of disease:
A. Ecological
B. Psychosocial
C. Biomedical
D. Holistic

139. The physical quality of life index consolidates all these, *except:*
A. Infant mortality
B. Life expectancy at age one
C. Literacy
D. Morbidity

140. Unit of rural planning and development is:
A. Block
B. Taluk
C. Corporation
D. District

141. The well in which the water rises the level of ground water:
A. Tube well
B. Step well
C. Dug well
D. Artesian well

142. The well taps the water from the above first impervious layer:
A. Shallow well
B. Deep well
C. Sanitary well
D. Artesian well

143. An instrument that measures the air velocity:
A. Anemometer
B. Barometer
C. Cyclometer
D. Psychrometer

---

135 A 136 D 137 A 138 C 139 D 140 A 141 D
142 A 143 A

144. Cyclops is the intermediate host of:
A. Ascariasis
B. Amoebiasis
C. Drancunculiasis
D. Ancylostomiasis

145. An animal associated with viral encephalitis:
A. Dog
B. Pig
C. Cat
D. Fox

146. The stage in which there is low birth and low death rate:
A. Early expanding
B. High stationary
C. Declining
D. Low stationary

147. Pulse polio immunization is given to:
A. Prevent polio
B. Eradicate polio
C. Reduce polio incidence
D. None of these

148. The first country that launched a nation-wide family planning programme:
A. China
B. Pakistan
C. England
D. India

149. The international health regulation is done by:
A. UNO
B. WHO
C. ILO
D. FAO

150. The heart of the slow sand filter:
A. Vital layer
B. Sand bed
C. Water level
D. Brick layer

151. Duration of immunity is long in:
A. Killed vaccine
B. Toxoids
C. Mixed vaccine
D. Live vaccine

152. Estimated fluid deficit in severe dehydration:
A. 40 to 50 ml/kg
B. 100 to 110 ml/kg
C. 50 to 75 ml/kg
D. 75 to 100 ml/kg

153. In India health for all by 2000 AD has been achieved through:
A. Comprehensive health care
B. Holistic health care
C. Primary health care
D. Community development programme

---

144 C 145 B 146 D 147 B 148 D 149 B 150 A
151 D 152 B 153 C

154. **Voluntary health agency involved actively in relief work is:**
A. Bharat Sevak Samaj
B. Indian Red Cross Society
C. Kasthurba Memorial Fund
D. Central Social Welfare Board

155. **The death of foetus in womb is called:**
A. Term birth
B. Abortion
C. Still birth
D. Miscarriage

156. **The recommended national target of trained dais to population in rural areas is:**
A. 1 : 2000
B. 1 : 500
C. 1 : 5000
D. 1 : 1000

157. **The growth chart recommended by Government of India has:**
A. Three reference curves
B. Two reference curves
C. Four reference curves
D. One reference curve

158. **National iodine deficiency disorders control programme was initiated by:**
A. Ministry of Health and Family Welfare
B. Ministry of Health and Social Welfare
C. Ministry of Social Welfare
D. Ministry of Education

159. **The most important tool for a community health worker is:**
A. Health education
B. Medication
C. Delivery kit
D. Job description

160. **Duration of maternity benefit according to ESI Act is:**
A. 30 days
B. 8 weeks
C. 12 weeks
D. 14 weeks

161. **The most appropriate time for IUD insertion is:**
A. During or within 10 days of menstruation
B. At about midst of the cycle
C. Just after menstruation
D. At any time of menstrual cycle

---

154 B 155 C 156 D 157 C 158 A 159 A 160 C
161 A

162. **The basic anthropometric measurements observed in infants are:**
   A. Height, weight, midarm circumference
   B. Height, weight, head circumference and chest circumference
   C. Height, weight, midarm circumference, head and chest circumference
   D. Weight, head and chest circumference

163. **Length of the baby at birth is about:**
   A. 25 cm
   B. 50 cm
   C. 60 cm
   D. 75 cm

164. **Bitot spot is caused by the deficiency of:**
   A. Vitamin B_1
   B. Vitamin B_6
   C. Vitamin A
   D. Vitamin B_{12}

165. **A rich source of iron is:**
   A. Green leaves
   B. Egg
   C. Milk
   D. Pulses

166. **Sanitary wells should be located:**
   A. 200 feet away from sewage
   B. 250 feet away from sewage
   C. 100 feet away from sewage
   D. 150 feet away from sewage

167. **The quantity of bleaching powder required to disinfect a well is:**
   A. 2 gms for 1000 litres of water
   B. 2.5 gms for 1000 litres of water
   C. 3 gms for 1000 litres of water
   D. 3.5 gms for 1000 litres of water

168. **Sewage purification takes place by the action of:**
   A. Aerobic organisms
   B. Anaerobic organisms
   C. Aerobic and anaerobic organisms
   D. None of the above

---

162 C 163 B 164 C 165 A 166 A 167 B 168 C

169. Innate immunity is the immunity the individual possesses by virtue of his:
A. Genetic make-up
B. As a result of previous infections
C. Introducing readymade antibodies into the body
D. None of the above

170. Concurrent disinfection means disinfecting the infectious agent:
A. Throughout the course of illness
B. After recovery from illness
C. After death of the sick person
D. During the pre-pathogenic phase

171. The antenatal mother need to be registered:
A. Before 12 weeks of pregnancy
B. Before 16 weeks of pregnancy
C. Before 10 weeks of pregnancy
D. As early as the pregnancy is diagnosed

172. Breast feeding needs to be initiated:
A. After 2 hours of delivery
B. After 3 days of delivery
C. After 2 days of delivery
D. Soon after birth

173. Rooming-in practice means:
A. Baby is kept in a separate room
B. Baby is kept close to the mother
C. Baby is kept in a warm room
D. Baby is kept in a nursery

174. Oral pill is not given to a lady when she is:
A. Menstruating
B. Breast feeding
C. Bleeding
D. None of the above

175. Poor man's meat is:
A. Ragi
B. Jowar
C. Pulses
D. Wheat

169 A 170 A 171 A 172 D 173 B 174 B 175 C

176. **A disease which is prevalent in a geographic area continuously at a low level is known as:**
   A. Epidemic
   B. Endemic
   C. Exotic
   D. Pandemic

177. **Retrospective studies is based on:**
   A. Present observations
   B. Past data or events
   C. Experiments
   D. None of the above

178. **Live vaccines are prepared from:**
   A. Live attenuated organisms
   B. Dead organism
   C. Live organism
   D. None of the above

179. **Pulse polio immunization gives:**
   A. Herd immunity
   B. Passive immunity
   C. Active immunity
   D. Acquired immunity

180. **The instrument used to measure the thermal comfort is:**
   A. Clinical thermometer
   B. Dial thermometer
   C. Kata thermometer
   D. Bath thermometer

181. **Measles is transmitted by:**
   A. Droplet infection
   B. Cross infection
   C. Direct contact
   D. Orofaecal route

182. **A latrine which is sanitary is the:**
   A. Water-seal latrine
   B. Pit latrine
   C. Bore hole latrine
   D. None of the above

---

176 D 177 B 178 A 179 C 180 C 181 A 182 A

183. The health survey and development committee was chaired by:
A. M.S. Chadah B. A.L. Mudaliar
C. A.K. Mukerji D. Joseph Bhore

184. Vitamin A is:
A. Water soluble B. Fat soluble
C. Both A and B D. None of the above

185. National malaria control programme came into force in the year:
A. 1953 B. 1954
C. 1958 D. 1957

186. The weight of a baby at birth is about:
A. 2 kg B. 2.5 kg
C. 3 kg D. 3.5 cm

187. November 14th is celebrated as:
A. Father's day B. Teacher's day
C. Children's day D. Elder's day

188. Causative organism for Koch's disease is:
A. M. tuberculo`sis B. M. leprae
C. M. diphtheriae D. None of the above

189. The causative organism for leprosy is:
A. M. leprae B. M. tuberculosis
C. Leprosy parasite D. None of the above

190. The health survey and planning committee was appointed in the year:
A. 1962 B. 1958
C. 1959 D. 1960

191. Babies born between 28th to 37th week are:
A. Full term babies B. Term babies
C. Post term babies D. Preterm babies

192. The postnatal period is also known as:
A. Antenatal period B. Intranatal period
C. Puerperium D. All the above

---

183 D 184 B 185 A 186 C 187 C 188 A 189 A
190 C 191 D 192 C

193. **The First Five Year Plan was started in:**
   A. 1947 B. 1949
   C. 1955 D. 1951

194. **Deficiency of iodine can cause:**
   A. Goitre B. Blindness
   C. Pellagra D. All the above

195. **Measles vaccine is given at the age of:**
   A. Birth B. 10 weeks
   C. Nine months D. 1 year

196. **April 7th is celebrated as:**
   A. World Population Day
   B. World Health Day
   C. International Nurse's Day
   D. World Women's Day

197. **Founder of the Red Cross movement:**
   A. Henry Durrant B. Robert Powell
   C. Joseph John D. None of the above

198. **Vaccines should be stored at a temperature of:**
   A. 0 C B. 8^{+} C
   C. 2 to 8 C D. Room temperature

199. **Whooping cough is also called as:**
   A. Pertusis B. Variolla
   C. Rubella D. Mumps

200. **The drug of choice in leprosy is:**
   A. Cotrimoxazole
   B. Dapsone
   C. Penicillin group
   D. All the above

201. **Birth weight of a newborn doubles at:**
   A. 3 months B. 6 months
   C. 9 months D. 1 year

202. **Birth weight of newborn triples at:**
   A. 3 months B. 6 months
   C. 9 months D. 1 year

---

193 D 194 A 195 C 196 B 197 A 198 C
199 A 200 B 201 B 202 D

203. Birth weight of newborn four times at:
A. 3 months B. 6 months
C. 1 year D. 2 years

204. Measles, mumps and rubella (MMR) vaccine is administered at the age of:
A. 6 months B. 12 months
C. 15 months D. 18 months

205. Measles vaccine is to be given at the end of:
A. 6 months B. 7 months
C. 8 months D. 9 months

206. Complete head control is achieved by:
A. 3–4 months B. 6–8 months
C. 7–9 months D. 4–6 months

207. Infant mortality rate is denoted per:
A. 1,000 live births B. 100 live births
C. 10,000 live birth D. None of these

208. Anterior fontanel closes by:
A. 9 months B. 12 months
C. 18 months D. 20 months

209. Folic acid deficiency during pregnancy can cause:
A. Cardiac anomaly B. Neural tube defect
C. Down syndrome D. Anomaly of brain

210. Newborn should be breastfed:
A. Every hourly B. On demand
C. Anytime D. Every 2nd hourly

211. Bacillus Calmette-Guerin (BCG) is a:
A. Live attenuated vaccine
B. Killed vaccine
C. Live vaccine
D. Toxoids

212. The incubation period of hepatitis B is:
A. 5–10 days B. 15–45 days
C. 45–60 days D. 60–90 days

---

203 D 204 C 205 D 206 A 207 A 208 C
209 B 210 B 211 A 212 A

213. **Dosage of vitamin A prophylaxis for children below 1 year is:**
A. 1 lakh IU
B. 2 lakh IU
C. 3 lakh IU
D. 5 lakh IU

214. **An illness transmitted through direct contact is:**
A. Typhoid
B. Hepatitis A
C. Human immunodeficiency virus/acquired immunodeficiency syndrome HIV/AIDS
D. Tuberculosis

215. **The first step in the control of communicable disease is:**
A. Notification
B. Isolation
C. Quarantine
D. Treatment

216. **Triple vaccine is:**
A. BCG
B. DPT
C. OPV
D. MMR

217. **The number of stages in the demographic cycle is:**
A. 2 B. 3
C. 4 D. 5

218. **Dracunliasis is a disease of:**
A. Vectorborne
B. Airborne
C. Waterborne
D. Foodborne

219. **German measles is otherwise called:**
A. Mumps
B. Rubella
C. Smallfox
D. Measles

220. **One of the waterborne disease is:**
A. Cholera
B. Malaria
C. Sexually transmitted disease STD
D. Tuberculosis TB

221. **An air pollutant that causes lung cancer is:**
A. Lead
B. Sulfur dioxide
C. Nitrogen
D. Hydrocarbons

---

213 A 214 C 215 B 216 B 217 D 218 C 219 B
220 A 221 D

222. **Incubation period for tetanus is:**
   A. 6–10 days
   B. 30 days
   C. 1 year
   D. 7–21 days

223. **It means the eligibility to bear children:**
   A. Eligible couple
   B. Vulnerable couple
   C. Target couple
   D. Married couple

224. **Following are the components of Reproductive and child Health RCH programme except:**
   A. Child survival and safe motherhood
   B. Prevention and management of reproductive tract infection RTI/STD/AIDS
   C. Client approach to health care
   D. Adolescent health

225. **The primary goal of essential newborn care is to reduce:**
   A. Neonatal mortality
   B. Perinatal and neonatal mortality
   C. Infant mortality
   D. All of the above

226. **The first dose of vitamin A is given at:**
   A. 6th month
   B. 9th month
   C. 8th month
   D. 10th month

227. **Currently International united nations international children's emergency fund UNICEF is promoting a campaign known as:**
   A. GOBI
   B. GOBIN
   C. GOBIFF
   D. GOBIF

228. **Solid wastes include all the following except:**
   A. Garbage
   B. Rubbish
   C. Demolished products
   D. Night soil

229. **Combined disposal of refuse and night soil is:**
   A. Composting
   B. Dumping
   C. Burial
   D. Incineration

230. **An example for primitive reflex is:**
   A. Grasping
   B. Crying
   C. Sneezing
   D. Coughing

---

222 A 223 A 224 C 225 D 226 B 227 C 228 D
229 A 230 A

231. **The shape of the anterior fontanel is:**
   A. Triangular
   B. Diamond
   C. Square
   D. Circular

232. **An infant born before the completion of 37 weeks of gestation is:**
   A. Postmature
   B. Premature
   C. Full term
   D. Large for gestational age

233. **Baby friendly hospital initiative was initiated by:**
   A. WHO
   B. UNICEF
   C. WHO and UNICEF
   D. FAO

234. **The one that protects against sexually transmitted diseases is:**
   A. Oral pills
   B. Intrauterine device IUD
   C. Condom
   D. Norplant

235. **Dichloro-diphenyl-trichloroethane (DDT) is a common:**
   A. Fungicide
   B. Insecticide
   C. Rodenticide
   D. Weedicide

236. **Beriberi is due to deficiency of:**
   A. Vitamin A
   B. Vitamin B1
   C. Vitamin C
   D. Vitamin B6

237. **Pyridoxine is the chemical name of:**
   A. Vitamin B2
   B. Vitamin B6
   C. Vitamin B12
   D. Vitamin K

238 **Embryonic period refers to the first:**
   A. 2 weeks
   B. 4 weeks
   C. 8 weeks
   D. 12 weeks

239 **In marasmus, there is lack of nutrients in:**
   A. Quantity
   B. Quality
   C. Both
   D. None

240 **In marasmus, the child looks like:**
   A. Healthy
   B. Oldman
   C. Active
   D. Playful

---

231 B **232** B **233** C **234** C **235** B **236** B **237** B
238 A **239** C **240** B

241 **Eruption of primary teeth is completed by:**
A. 18 months B. 24 months
C. 30 months D. 36 months

242 **Toilet training is the main task during:**
A. Infant B. Toddler
C. Preschool D. School going

243 **Loss of birth weight within 10 days after birth is:**
A. 10% B. 15%
C. 25% D. 30%

244 **The neonate is considered as term baby at the ___ weeks of gestation.**
A. 32 weeks B. 34 weeks
C. 36 weeks D. 38 weeks

245 **Exclusive breastfeeding to be given up to:**
A. 3 months B. 4 months
C. 6 months D. 8 months

246 **Physiological jaundice appear after birth:**
A. 1–2 days B. 3–4 days
C. 5–6 days D. Above 1 week

247 **Physiological jaundice will disappear within:**
A. 7 days B. 10 days
C. 15 days D. > 15 days

248. **Pathological jaundice is within:**
A. 24 hours B. 36 hours
C. 48 hours D. > 48 hours

249. **Pathological jaundice persists beyond:**
A. 1 week B. 2 weeks
C. 1 month D. 2 months

250. **The physiological jaundice in preterm baby disappears at:**
A. 1 week B. 2 weeks
C. 4 weeks D. > 4 weeks

---

241 D 242 B 243 A 244 D 245 C 246 A 247 A
248 A 249 B 250 B

251. **Parallel play is seen in:**
A. Infant
B. Toddler
C. Prescholar
D. Scholage

252. **The major feature of severe marasmus is:**
A. Edema
B. Severe loss of subcutaneous fat
C. Sparse hair
D. Dry skin

253. **Anganwadi workers are part of:**
A. Balwadi scheme
B. Integrated child development scheme (ICDS)
C. Project scheme
D. National scheme

254. **An infant with less than 2.5 kg birth weight inrespective of gestational age is known as:**
A. Preterm
B. Term
C. Small fordate
D. Low birth weight

255. **Common mode of transmission of hookworm is:**
A. Skin penetration
B. Hand to mouth
C. Water
D. Air

256. **The one measures the death of women due to puerperal causes is:**
A. Maternal mortality
B. Perinatal mortality
C. Natal mortality
D. All of these

257. **If the ovum is fertilized by the sperm carrying X chromosome, the result is:**
A. Female offspring
B. Male offspring
C. Twins
D. Deformed offspring

258. **If the ovum is fertilized by the sperm carrying Y chromosome the result is:**
A. Female offspring
B. Male offspring
C. Twins
D. Deformed offspring

---

251 B 252 B 253 B 254 C 255 A 256 A 257 A
258 B

259. Expected date of delivery (EDD) is calculated from the last menstrual period (LMP) by:
A. Adding 7 days and counting 9 months forward
B. Adding 7 days and counting 8 months forward
C. Adding 7 days and counting 10 months forward
D. None of these

260. A mother gives her LMP as February 2nd, 2010; her EDD is:
A. November 6th, 2010
B. November 7th, 2010
C. November 8th, 2010
D. November 9th, 2010

261. The placenta transports nutrients and oxygen to the fetus by:
A. Osmosis
B. Diffusion
C. Gravitation
D. None of those

262. Colostrum can be expressed from the breast from the weeks of:
A. 12
B. 16
C. 20
D. 24

263. The first fetal movement felt by the mother is called:
A. Lightening
B. Quickening
C. Moving
D. Molding

264. Nullipara means, a woman who has:
A. Never been pregnant
B. First time pregnant
C. Pregnant after long time
D. Not produced a viable child

265. Primipara means, a woman who has:
A. First time pregnant
B. Never been pregnant
C. Pregnant more than once
D. Not produced a viable child

266. Mrs R had three pregnancy in which she had one live birth, one stillbirth and one abortion. Her classification is:
A. G3 P3 L1 SB1 A1
B. G3 P1 SB1 A1 L1
C. G3 P2 SB1 A1 LB1
D. G3 P2 LB SB2 A1 L1

---

259 A 260 D 261 C 262 D 263 B 264 D
265 A 266 A

267. **The hormone responsible for the production of milk is:**
    A. Oxytocin B. Estrogen
    C. Progesterone D. Prolactin

268. **The posterior fortanel closes:**
    A. Soon after birth B. 6 months after birth
    C. 1 year after birth D. 1½ year after birth

269. **The vaginal discharge during postpartum period is called:**
    A. Menstruation B. Lochia
    C. Lanngo D. Discharge

270. **The normal length of an umbilical cord is:**
    A. 25 cm B. 50 cm
    C. 75 cm D. 100 cm

271. **Poliomyelitis is caused by:**
    A. RNA virus B. DNA virus
    C. Myxovirus D. Epstein-Barr (EB) virus

272. **Sabin vaccine is otherwise known as:**
    A. DPT B. OPV
    C. Typhoid vaccine D. DV (Diphtheria vaccine)

273. **The causative agent for acute diarrheal disease in children is:**
    A. Enterovirus B. Astrovirus
    C. Rotavirus D. Coronavirus

274. **The mode of transmission of typhoid fever is:**
    A. Direct B. Airborne
    C. Waterborne D. Vectorborne

275. **The composition of atmospheric air includes nitrogen, oxygen and:**
    A. Carbon dioxide B. Carbon monoxide
    C. Hydrogen sulfide D. Sulpher dioxide

276. **Atmospheric air self, cleaning mechanism is by:**
    A. Chemical charge B. Respiration
    C. Wind D. Fumes

---

267 A 268 A 269 B 270 B 271 A 272 B 273 C
274 C 275 A 276 C

277. The body mass index (BMI) of an individual 30–39.9 denotes:
A. Underweight B. Overweight
C. Obese D. Morbidly obese

278. Legal age of marriage for girls is:
A. 15 years B. 18 years
C. 20 years D. 22 years

279. An example for the chemical method of contraception is:
A. Condom B. Jellies
C. Pills D. Cervical cap

280. An example for the hormonal method of contraception is:
A. Condom B. Foam
C. Pills D. Vault

281. Vault is an example for method of contraception:
A. Physical B. Chemical
C. Hormonal D. None of these

282. An example for third generation intrauterine device is:
A. Lippe's loop B. Copper T
C. Norplant D. Progestasert

283. Papanicolaou smear is done to rule out:
A. Ca uterus B. Ca vagina
C. Ca cervix D. All of these

284. Norplant is a:
A. Male pill B. Female pill
C. Implant D. IUD

285. The number of females per 1,000 males is:
A. Sex ratio B. Family ratio
C. Literacy ratio D. Age pyramid

286. The number of live births per 1,000 divided by mid year population is:
A. Birth rate B. Fertility rate
C. Total fertility rate D. Total population rate

277 B 278 B 279 B 280 C 281 A 202 B 283 C
284 C 285 A 286 A

287. **The one used as an indicator of human development is:**
A. Life expectancy
B. Literacy
C. Sex ratio
D. Growth

288. **Absolute or relative lack of nutrient produce:**
A. Under nutrition
B. Over nutrition
C. Deficiency
D. Imbalance

289. **The first Five Year Plan was started during the period of:**
A. 1946–1951
B. 1951–56
C. 1956–61
D. 1961–66

290. **Addressing the unmet needs of contraception, personnel and infrastructure is the objective of:**
A. National Health Policy
B. Five Year Plan
C. National Population Policy
D. National Educational Policy

291. **Health service to every 5,000 population is provided through:**
A. Subcenter
B. Primary health centre
C. Community health center
D. Taluk hospital

292. **Health service that links all other health services is:**
A. Referral service
B. Transfer service
C. Ambulance service
D. Outpatient service

293. **The one that governs the urban area of more than 1 lakh population is:**
A. Panchayat
B. Town Panchayat
C. Municipality
D. Corporation

294. **The following are the mass level approaches of health education except:**
A. Cinema
B. Television
C. Radio
D. E-mail

---

287 A 288 C 289 A 290 C 291 A 292 A 293 D
294 D

295. The calorie and protein requirement provided through the Midday Meal is:

A. 1/3 calorie, ½ protein
B. ½ calorie, 1/3 protein
C. ½ calorie, ½ protein
D. 1/3 calorie, protein

296. Siderosis is the occupational disease caused by:

A. Silica
B. Iron
C. Asbestos
D. Cotton

297. The occupational disease caused by hay or pollen dust inhalation is:

A. Bagossis
B. Byssinosis
C. Asbestosis
D. Farmer's lung

298. The vector responsible for filarial fever is:

A. Mosquito
B. Fly
C. Flea
D. Rodent

299. Mode of transmission for swineflu is:

A. Droplet
B. Water
C. Vector
D. Air

300. Number of iron tablets to be taken by an antenatal mother during pregnancy is:

A. 50
B. 100
C. 150
D. 200

301. Pioneer of community health nursing is:

A. Lillian wald
B. Hildegard
C. Florence
D. Calister

302. The fore runner of the sanitary latrine is:

A. Bore hole
B. Dug wall
C. Research cum action (RCA)
D. Planning, research and action Institute (PRAI)

303. Water seal in a sanitary latrine is provided by

A. Pan
B. Trap
C. Connecting pipe
D. Squatting plate

---

295 C 296 B 297 D 298 A 299 D 300 B 301 A
302 A 303 B

304. **In the burial ground, trees are planted to absorb:**
A. Nitric acid
B. Sulfuric acid
C. Carbonic acid
D. Hydrochloric acid

305. **Garbage is the:**
A. Food wastes
B. Plastic wastes
C. Sewage
D. Dead animals

306. **Disposal of refuse and night soil is by:**
A. Dumping
B. Composting
C. Burning
D. Burging

307. **Kitchen waste water is called as:**
A. Sewage
B. Sullage
C. Effluent
D. Liquid waste

308. **Industrial waste is called:**
A. Sewage
B. Sullage
C. Effluent
D. Waste

309. **Transmission of fecal borne diseases is by all except:**
A. Water
B. Flies
C. Food
D. Air

310. **Social security to general population is:**
A. Employee's State Insurance (ESI) benefit
B. Insurance
C. Pension
D. None

311. **Social security provided to general population is:**
A. Insurance
B. Pension
C. Police security
D. None

312. **Social security provided to public servants is:**
A. Insurance
B. Pension
C. Police security
D. None

313. **Varicella – Zoster is the causative organism for:**
A. Smallpox
B. Chickenpox
C. Measles
D. Mumps

304 C 305 A 306 B 307 B 308 C 309 D 310 B
311 C 312 B 313 B

314. As per Universal Immunization Program (UIP) measles vaccine is given at:

A. 9th month B. End of 9th month

C. 10th month D. 11th month

315. Vaccine that prevents triple diseases is:

A. OPV B. BCG

C. MMR D. DT

316. Hepatitis infection was formerly known as:

A. Delta hepatitis B. Serum hepatitis

C. Infections hepatitis D. Jaundice

317. Presence of rice water stool is the specific indicator of:

A. Typhoid B. Cholera

C. Amebiasis D. Dysentry

318. The vector responsible to transmit dengue fever is:

A. Mosquito B. Fly

C. Tich D. Rodent

319. The following are the surface infections except:

A. Trachoma B. Leprosy

C. Tuberculosis D. Tetanus

320. In demographic cycle, the stage characterized by a low birth and low death rate is:

A. Early expanding B. Late expanding

C. Low stationary D. High stationary

321. The killing power of one specific disease is:

A. Death rate B. Case fatality

C. Morbidity rate D. Incidence rate

322. Any departure, subjective or objective from a state of physiological well-being is defined to be:

A. Mortality B. Morbidity

C. Incidence D. Prevalence

---

314 B 315 C 316 D 317 B 318 A 319 D 320 C
321 B 322 B

323. The science and art of preventing disease, prolonging life and promoting health and efficiency through organized effort is:
A. Community health
B. Family health
C. Individual health
D. Social health

324. Uncovering health needs and problems through observation interviews and records is:
A. Assessment
B. Planning
C. Implementation
D. Evaluation

325. The nurse shares information on purpose for home visit with family during:
A. Pre-visit phase
B. Visit phase
C. Post visit phase
D. Termination phase

326. Problems of home visit are:
A. Assessment and implementation
B. Non-acceptance and role confusion
C. Saving time and energy
D. Early identification of health problems

327. The continuous scrutiny of all aspects of occurrence and spread of disease is:
A. Epidemiology
B. Community health
C. Surveillance
D. Monitoring

328. The one not present in surveillance cycle is:
A. Collection of data
B. Analysis of data
C. Monitoring the data
D. Disseminating the data

329. The raw material of the surveillance system is:
A. Incidence
B. Data
C. Prevalence
D. Message

330. The second stage of the natural history of the disease is:
A. Prepathogenesis
B. Pathogenesis
C. Postpathogenesis
D. None of these

---

323 A 324 A 325 B 326 B 327 C 328 C 329 D
330 B

331. The first stage of the natural history of the disease is:
A. Prepathogenesis
B. Pathogenesis
C. Postpathogenesis
D. None of these

332. Incidence rate is defined as:
A. Number of old cases occurring in a defined population
B. Number of new cases occurring in a defined population
C. Number of new and old cases occurring in a defined population
D. None of the above

333. Disease prevalence refers to:
A. Number of old cases occurring in a defined population
B. Number of new cases occurring in a defined population
C. Number of new and old cases occurring in a defined population
D. None of the above

334. Postcoital contraception is recommended to take within ...... hours of unprotected intercourse:
A. 24 hours
B. 48 hours
C. 72 hours
D. One week

335. The indicator of prevalence of contraceptive practice in the community is:
A. Total fertility rate
B. Net reproduction rate
C. Gross reproduction rate
D. Couple protection rate

336. Second generation of IUD is:
A. Non-medicated IUD
B. Copper IUD
C. Lippes loop
D. Hormone-releasing IUD

337. First generation of IUD is:
A. Non-medicated IUD
B. Copper IUD
C. Lippes loop
D. Hormone-releasing IUD

338. Third generation of IUD is:
A. Non-medicated IUD
B. Copper IUD
C. Lippes loop
D. Hormone-releasing IUD

331 A 332 B 333 C 334 C 335 D 336 A 337 C
338 B

339. **The global indicator of adequacy of growth of children is:**
   A. Birth weight
   B. Weight for age
   C. Height for age
   D. Head circumference

340. **Vaccine contraindicated for a newborn with HIV is:**
   A. OPV
   B. BCG
   C. Hepatitis B
   D. All of these

341. **The central triangle in under-five symbol indicates:**
   A. Care in illness
   B. Immunization
   C. Growth monitoring
   D. Family planning

342. **The backbone of all maternal and child health (MCH) services except:**
   A. Antenatal care
   B. Postnatal care
   C. Neonatal care
   D. Illness care

343. **The most important indication of health status of a community is:**
   A. Maternal mortality rate
   B. Infant mortality rate
   C. Death rate
   D. Postneonatal mortality rate

344. **Patients receiving isoniazid (INH) are supplemented with 10 mg/day of:**
   A. Pyridoxine
   B. Riboflavin
   C. Folate
   D. All

345. **All the following inhibit iron absorption except:**
   A. Phyrates in bran
   B. Phosphates in egg yolk
   C. Tannin and tea
   D. Ascarbic acid in guava

346. **The following cancers are due to risk of occupational except:**
   A. Skin cancer
   B. Lung cancer
   C. Bladder cancer
   D. Leukemia

---

339 B 340 B 341 D 342 D 343 B 344 A 345 D
346 D

347. Components of RCH programme are Child survival and safe motherhood (CSSM), STD and:

A. ICDS

B. OBFIH

O: Oral hydration

B: Breastfeeding

F: Family planning

I: Immunization

H: Health education

C. RTI (Reproductive tract infection)

D. None of these

348. Keeping the baby by the side of the mother is called:

A. Rooming-in
B. Newborn care
C. Kangaroo care
D. Nutritional care

349. DOTS is:

A. Directly observed treatment scheme
B. Directly observed treatment system
C. Directly observed therapy scheme
D. Directly Observed Treatment Short course

350. One block consists of:

A. 50 village
B. 100 villages
C. 150 villages
D. 125 villages

351. The test for pasteurized milk is:

A. Phosphatase test
B. Orthotolidine test
C. Ochratoxin A (OTA) test
D. Albumin test

352. The disease which is not transmitted by eating wholesome meat is:

A. Tinea solium
B. Tinea saginata
C. Anthrax
D. Q fever

353. The food standards set by the Directorate of Marketing and Inspection, Government of India is:

A. Prevention of Food Adulteration (PFA)
B. Agmark
C. ISD
D. Codex

347 A 348 A 349 A 350 B 351 A 352 D 353 B

354. The ideal candidate for IUD insertion are the following except:

A. Nulliparas
B. No history of pelvic inflammatory disease (PID)
C. Has normal periods
D. Willing to check the IUD tail

355. The cheap and best sources of iron is:

A. Beatroot B. Green leaves
C. Jaggery D. Rice

356. Egg contains all vitamins except:

A. Vitamin A B. Vitamin B
C. Vitamin C D. Vitamin D

357. Vitamin C deficiency is:

A. Beriberi B. Scurvy
C. Night blindness D. Stomatitis

358. A complete protein from vegetarian diet is:

A. Soyabeans B. Moong
C. Ragi D. Rice

359. Planned visit to the family is:

A. Clinical visit B. Home visit
C. Community visit D. Center visit

360. The following diseases are by vehicle borne transmission except:

A. Polio B. Cholera
C. Worms infestation D. STD

361. The following morbidity rates are used for assessing health status in the community except:

A. Incidence
B. Prevalence
C. Disability adjusted life year
D. Duration of hospital stay

362. Transfer of antibodies through placenta is an example for ______ immunity:

A. Active B. Passive
C. Herd D. Cellular

---

354 A **355** B **356** C **357** B **358** A **359** B **360** D
361 D **362** B

363. Slate-colored spots on buttocks of newborn is called as:
A. Mangolian spot
B. Stroke bites
C. Erythema
D. Echymosis

364. Frequent occurrence of masturbation is seen in:
A. School going
B. Preschooler
C. Preadolescent
D. Adolescent

365. First level of health is taken care off by:
A. Primary health center
B. Taluk hospital
C. District hospital
D. Teaching hospital

366. The color of stools in breastfed infants is:
A. Yellowish brown
B. Greenish brown
C. Pale yellow
D. Yellow

367. Following vasectomy, the couple has to follow contraception till:
A. 6 weeks after surgery
B. 3 months after surgery
C. One sperm count test to be negative
D. Two sperms count to be negative

368. Pregnant mother should avoid taking any drug to prevent:
A. Nausea/Vomiting
B. Abortion
C. Teratogenic effect
D. Side effects of drugs

369. Prenatal mortality combines all of the following except:
A. Fetal death after 28 weeks of gestation
B. Death during labor
C. Death within 7 days of birth
D. Death after 7 days of birth

370. In calculating fertility rate, when only married woman are considered, it is known as:
A. General marital fertility rate
B. Total fertility rate
C. Net reproduction rate
D. Gross reproduction rate

363 A 364 D 365 A 366 B 367 D 368 C 369 D
370 A

371. Active participation in meeting the needs of health needs is the purpose of:

A. Home visit
B. Clinic visit
C. Hospital visit
D. Personal visit

372. 0–28 days from the day of birth of child belongs to the period of:

A. Neonatal
B. Infancy
C. Toddler
D. Natal

373. Newborn is at risk of:

A. Hypothermia
B. Dehydration
C. Hyperthermia
D. Hypotention

374. A reliable indicator of the health status of children is:

A. Infant mortality
B. Neonatal mortality
C. Natal mortality
D. Maternal mortality

375. Constituted BCG vaccine should be used within:

A. 24 hours
B 12 hours
C. 6 hours
D. 3 hours

---

371 A 372 A 373 A 374 A 375 B

CHAPTER 3

Nursing Education

1. **One of 3 languages for communicating information about quantities is:**
   A. Graphic representative B. Models
   C. Specimen D. Over-head projection

2. **A teaching material that stimulate some life object is:**
   A. Mock-up B. Moulage
   C. Models D. An object

3. **The criteria used for selecting evaluation devices all, *except:***
   A. Validity B. Reliability
   C. Practicality D. Complementary

4. **The best one that is used in teaching to show a equipment which is difficult to have in a classroom is:**
   A. Projected aids B. Non-projected aids
   C. Three dimensional aids D. All of these

5. **Multiple aspects of the topic is discussed in:**
   A. Seminar B. Symposium
   C. Workshop D. Conference

6. **A one that helps the student teacher to acquire teaching skills in a simplified manner is:**
   A. Macro teaching B. Micro teaching
   C. Classroom teaching D. Clinical teaching

7. **The blueprint of nursing care rendered to a patient by a nursing student is:**
   A. Nursing care study
   B. Nursing care plan
   C. Family care study
   D. Teach care plan

---

1 A 2 B 3 D 4 C 5 A 6 B 7 B

8. **A one that is very flexible without rigid rules, regulations and fixed stages is:**
   A. Formal education
   B. Non-formal education
   C. Informal education
   D. Continuing education

9. **Indian Nursing Council was established in the year:**
   A. 1945
   B. 1947
   C. 1949
   D. 1951

10. **Counselling is given in:**
    A. Informal setting
    B. Formal setting
    C. Both
    D. None

11. **The proponents of naturalism is:**
    A. Aristotle
    B. Plato
    C. John Dewey
    D. Ralph Taylar

12. **Learning that is carried out in the affective domain is:**
    A. Ideational learning
    B. Psychomotor learning
    C. Skill learning
    D. Passive learning

13. **An experience acquired through the use of words, written and oral, and other symbols is:**
    A. Direct experience
    B. Indirect experience
    C. Symbolic experience
    D. Vicarious experience

14. **The substantive dimension in the educative process refers to:**
    A. Syllabus
    B. Curriculum
    C. Institution
    D. Hospital

15. **Elements in the learning process are the following, *except:***
    A. Goal
    B. Response
    C. Integration
    D. Evaluation

16. **The curriculum that consists of the content planned by a teacher is:**
    A. Societal curriculum
    B. Institutional curriculum
    C. Hidden curriculum
    D. Instructional curriculum

---

8 C 9 A 10 A 11 A 12 B 13 C 14 B
15 D 16 D

17. **In India a financial year is from:**
A. May to April
B. June to May
C. April to March
D. March to Feb

18. **Presentation of a pre-arranged series of events to a group is:**
A. Debate
B. Demonstration
C. Discussion
D. Dissection

19. **Questioning helps to:**
A. Stimulate thinking
B. Evaluate
C. Fear the student
D. Obtain appraisal

20. **The vertical organization of learning experience refers to:**
A. Sequence
B. Continuity
C. Integration
D. Both A and B

21. **Learning is:**
A. Self active
B. Instructed
C. Forced
D. Perceived

22. **Emotional learning is termed as:**
A. Cognitive
B. Affective
C. Assimilative
D. Active

23. **Theology is the science of:**
A. Arts
B. Science
C. Medicine
D. God

24. **A revolt against traditional system of education was:**
A. Idealism
B. Realism
C. Naturalism
D. Pragmatism

25. **Repressive forgetting occurs as a result of factors related to:**
A. Past events
B. Outside the individual
C. Within the individual
D. Present events

26. **Indian Nursing Council Act was passed in the year:**
A. 1935
B. 1940
C. 1945
D. 1947

---

17 C 18 B 19 A 20 D 21 A 22 B 23 D
24 C 25 B 26 D

27. **Brain storming is a type of:**
    A. Role play
    B. Method of teaching
    C. Group interaction
    D. Workshop

28. **Mock-up means:**
    A. Specimen
    B. Cartoons
    C. Models
    D. Charts

29. **Successful education practices are based upon:**
    A. Psychological principles
    B. Evaluating techniques
    C. Teaching techniques
    D. Learning principles

30. **The one that helps to acquire characteristics of positive nature, such as self-control, etc is:**
    A. Education
    B. Learning
    C. Discipline
    D. Control

31. **Learning that is carried out in the cognitive domain is:**
    A. Ideational learning
    B. Skill learning
    C. Emotional learning
    D. Passive learning

32. **An experience acquired through the medium of A.V. Aids is:**
    A. Direct experience
    B. Vicarious experience
    C. Symbolic experience
    D. Indirect experience

33. **One form of graphic presentation is:**
    A. Poster
    B. Notice board
    C. Charts
    D. Black board

34. **A complete evaluation program includes all, *except:***
    A. Evaluation of educational objectives
    B. Evaluation of teaching and learning procedures
    C. Evaluation of student progress
    D. Evaluation of records

---

27 B 28 C 29 A 30 C 31 A 32 B 33 C
34 D

35. **Single aspect of the topic is discussed in:**
A. Symposium
B. Seminar
C. Workshop
D. Conference

36. **It is a teacher education technique which allows teachers to apply teaching skills:**
A. Macro teaching
B. Micro-teaching
C. Classroom teaching
D. Clinical teaching

37. **Oral examination provides:**
A. Flexibility
B. Direct control
C. Bias
D. All

38. **The standardized test includes all, *except:***
A. Aptitude test
B. Personality test
C. Prognostic test
D. Teacher made test

39. **Incentive used by the teacher is:**
A. Praise
B. Punishment
C. Imposition
D. Excuse

40. **Guidance is given in:**
A. Formal setting
B. Informal setting
C. Both
D. None

41. **ANM programme started in the year:**
A. 1940
B. 1941
C. 1942
D. 1943

42. **The father of idealism is:**
A. Gandhi
B. Socrates
C. Tagore
D. Plato

43. **Shiksha is the synonym of:**
A. Education
B. Curriculum
C. Discipline
D. Learner

44. **The one necessitates flexibility in designing the curriculum is the:**
A. Formal education
B. Informal education
C. Non-formal education
D. None of these

35 A 36 B 37 D 38 D 39 A 40 D 41 C
42 D 43 A 44 C

45. **Religious institution is an example for:**
    A. Informal agency
    B. Formal agency
    C. Active agency
    D. Passive agency

46. **Chairman of Secondary Education Commission was:**
    A. Dr. Kothari
    B. Dr. Radhakrishnan
    C. Dr. Bhare
    D. Dr. Mudaliar

47. **John dewey is the chief exponent of:**
    A. Realism
    B. Naturalism
    C. Pragmatism
    D. Idealism

48. **The founder and father of pragmatism is:**
    A. William James
    B. John Dewey
    C. Roussane
    D. Dalton

49. **Giving information and directing action is:**
    A. Guidance
    B. Advising
    C. Counselling
    D. Psychotherapy

50. **Finding further opportunities to serve qualified students is by:**
    A. Appraisal service
    B. Orientation service
    C. Followup service
    D. Counselling service

51. **Constitution of a curriculum preparation committee is a sub-step of:**
    A. Planning
    B. Implementation
    C. Evaluation
    D. Development

52. **Discussion on a particular topic by few members is the:**
    A. Panel discussion
    B. Seminar
    C. Symposium
    D. Workshop

53. **A device for displaying study material is the:**
    A. Felt board
    B. Bulletin board
    C. Flannel board
    D. Chalk board

54. **Criteria for selection of evaluative devices, *except:***
    A. Sampling course content
    B. Validity
    C. Reliability
    D. Acceptability

---

45 B 46 D 47 C 48 A 49 B 50 C 51 D
52 A 53 B 54 D

55. **Intrinsic programming was developed by:**
A. Skinner
B. Schramm
C. Crowder
D. Eigen

56. **The one emphasizes the functional relationship between the device and reality is:**
A. A model
B. A mockup
C. A moulage
D. A specimen

57. **An education where there is no specially qualified personnel to teach is a:**
A. Non-formal education
B. Informal education
C. Formal education
D. Continuing education

58. **The wide acceptance of the unit concept of learning was made by:**
A. Herbert
B. Morrison
C. John Dewey
D. Dalton

59. **Contiguous conditioning theory was made by:**
A. Tharndike
B. Hull
C. Guthrie
D. Tolman

60. **Law of preparedness is also called as:**
A. Law of readiness
B. Law of effect
C. Law of exercise
D. Law of belongingness

61. **University Education Commission was constituted in the year:**
A. 1964
B. 1952
C. 1948
D. 1950

62. **Curriculum planned by a faculty for a clearly identified group of students is:**
A. Societal curriculum
B. Instructional curriculum
C. Institutional curriculum
D. None of the above

63. **The excellent learning for a nursing student is:**
A. Team nursing
B. Patient assignment
C. Functional nursing
D. Night duty

---

55 C 56 B 57 B 58 B 59 C 60 A 61 C
62 C 63 B

64. **Lesson plan should be:**
   A. Teacher centered
   B. Subject centered
   C. Class centered
   D. Student centered

65. **Written report of conversation between nurse and patient is:**
   A. Process recording
   B. Progress recording
   C. Outcome recording
   D. Clinical recording

66. **Competition means:**
   A. Conflicting
   B. Compromising
   C. Moving above
   D. Comparing

67. **The purpose of teaching is to facilitate:**
   A. Acting
   B. Learning
   C. Practising
   D. Teaching

68. **Ambiguity of a question means:**
   A. Precise
   B. Double meaning
   C. Upto the point
   D. Very clean

69. **Three dimensional aids is:**
   A. Flip chart
   B. Overhead projection
   C. Specimen
   D. Tape recorder

70. **Tutoring means:**
   A. Good counselling
   B. Good guidance
   C. Good listening
   D. Subject centered

71. **One type of error in evaluation is:**
   A. Halo error
   B. Objectivity error
   C. Physical error
   D. Self activity error

72. **Mathein means:**
   A. Educate
   B. Learn
   C. Teach
   D. Explain

73. **Unit planning provides a sound basis for:**
   A. Planning
   B. Implementation
   C. Evaluation
   D. Replanning

74. **Concentration is the result of:**
   A. Motivation
   B. Perception
   C. Interest
   D. Control of attention

---

64 D 65 A 66 C 67 B 68 B 69 C 70 D
71 A 72 B 73 C 74 D

75. **Skill learning is carried out in the:**
A. Cognitive domain
B. Psychomotor domain
C. Affective domain
D. All

76. **Self enhancement is the philosophy of:**
A. Idealism
B. Naturalism
C. Realism
D. Neo-realism

77. **Pedagogy is the synonymous of:**
A. Curriculum
B. Education
C. Discipline
D. Learner

78. **An indirect, incidental and spontaneous one is the:**
A. Formal education
B. Non-formal education
C. Informal education
D. None of these

79. **Professional organization is the example for:**
A. Active agency
B. Passive agency
C. Formal agency
D. Informal agency

80. **Chairman of University Education Commission was:**
A. Dr. Mudaliar
B. Dr. Kothari
C. Dr. Nhare
D. Dr. Radhakrishnan

81. **The remedial activity belongs to:**
A. Guidance
B. Psychotherapy
C. Counselling
D. Advising

82. **Gathering adequate information about pupils is by:**
A. Appraisal service
B. Orientation service
C. Followup service
D. Counselling service

83. **Making key decision is a sub-step of:**
A. Evaluation
B. Implementation
C. Planning
D. Development

---

75 B 76 A 77 B 78 C 79 D 80 D 81 B
82 A 83 C

84. **Attitude of a student is assessed by:**
    A. Check list B. Rating scale
    C. Analogy D. Assignment

85. **Extrinsic programming was developed by:**
    A. Eigen B. Schramm
    C. Skinner D. Crowder

86. **A part of an object is the:**
    A. Chart B. Specimen
    C. Model D. Exhibit

87. **An experience acquired through the medium of A.V. Aids is:**
    A. Direct B. Indirect
    C. Vicarious D. Symbolic

88. **Four essentials in the learning process was stressed by:**
    A. Herbert B. John Dewey
    C. Dalton D. Morrison

89. **The curricula planned for a large group or class of students is the:**
    A. Core B. Individual
    C. Institutional D. Societal

90. **Law of habit formation is also called as:**
    A. Law of preparedness B. Law of effect
    C. Law of exercise D. Law of belongingness

91. **Systematic behaviour theory was given by:**
    A. Tolman B. Tharndike
    C. Hull D. Guthrie

92. **Kothari Education Commission was constituted in the year:**
    A. 1947-48 B. 1964-66
    C. 1952-53 D. 1960-62

93. **The synthesis or harmonious blend of the diverse philosophics of education is the:**
    A. Eclectism B. Neo-realism
    C. Existentialism D. Pragmatism

---

84 D 85 C 86 B 87 C 88 A 89 D 90 C
91 C 92 B 93 A

94. **The word education is derived from the word educare which is a:**
A. Greek work
B. German word
C. Latin word
D. None of these

95. **The word educare means:**
A. Bring up
B. Leadout
C. Train
D. Mould

96. **The term which is commonly used for mentioning education is:**
A. Postology
B. Philosophy
C. Pathology
D. Pedagogy

97. **The definition—education is the development of all those capacities in the individual which will enable him to control his environment and fulfill his possibilities—is given by:**
A. John Dewey
B. Pestalozzi
C. Socrates
D. Jhorndike

98. **In India, the first school of nursing was started in:**
A. Vellore
B. Delhi
C. Chennai
D. Mumbai

99. **Five branch of philosophy are follows *except:***
A. Axiology
B. Metaphysics
C. Emporiatic
D. Epistemology

100. **The one concerned with the systematic study of knowledge and its inter-relationship is:**
A. Axiology
B. Metaphysics
C. Logic
D. Aesthetics

101. **According to an idealist, the essence of life is:**
A. Material nature
B. Spiritual nature
C. Practical nature
D. Only nature

102. **The popular method of teaching namely kindergarten was developed by:**
A. Annie Besant
B. John Dewey
C. Froebal
D. Pluto

---

94 C 95 A 96 D 97 A 98 C 99 C 100 C
101 B 102 C

103. The philosophy that says, no need for a rigid curriculum is:
A. Idealism
B. Realism
C. Naturalism
D. Functionalism

104. Functionalism is the other name for:
A. Idealism
B. Realism
C. Naturalism
D. Pragmatism

105. Learning by doing was advocated by:
A. John Dewey
B. Pluto
C. Froebal
D. Annie Besant

106. Broad field curriculum is suggested by:
A. Pregmatist
B. Idealist
C. Naturalist
D. Realist

107. The one opposes bookish knowledge is:
A. Realism
B. Naturalism
C. Idealism
D. Pragmatism

108. Objective method of teaching is recommended by:
A. Realist
B. Idealist
C. Naturalist
D. Functionalist

109. Teleconferencing is a:
A. Formal education
B. Information education
C. Non-formal education
D. None of these

110. M. phil. programme in nursing was started first in:
A. Vellore
B. New Delhi
C. Mumbai
D. Kolkata

111. The one that depicts what the student should be able to do after the teaching-learning activity is:
A. Educational objective
B. Central objective
C. Behavioural objective
D. Instructional objective

---

103 C 104 D 105 A 106 A 107 A 108 D 109 C
110 B 111 A

112. Dynamic nature of education will be maintained by:
A. Realism
B. Pragmatism
C. Existentialism
D. Eclectism

113. The definition—Education is the allround drawing out the best in child and man—body, mind and spirit—is given by:
A. Dr. Radhakrishnan
B. Mahatma Gandhi
C. Annie Besant
D. Jakir Hussain

114. In India the first school of nursing was started in the year:
A. 1871
B. 1872
C. 1873
D. 1874

115. The one deals with the ultimate true nature of things is the:
A. Logic
B. Metaphysics
C. Aesthetics
D. Axiology

116. The one studies about the beauty and harmony in life is the:
A. Logic
B. Metaphysics
C. Aesthetics
D. Axiology

117. The one is concerned with the nature of morality and value is:
A. Logic
B. Metaphysics
C. Aesthetics
D. Axiology

118. Instrumentalism is the other name for:
A. Idealism
B. Realism
C. Naturalism
D. Pragmatism

119. Experimentalism is the other name for:
A. Idealism
B. Realism
C. Naturalism
D. Pragmatism

120. Philosophy is an attempt to think truly about human experience or to make out whole experience intelligible is the definition given by:
A. Brightman
B. Henderson
C. Raymond
D. Rousseau

---

112 D 113 B 114 A 115 B 116 C 117 D 118 D
119 D 120 A

121. **Philosophy is a search for comprehensive view of nature, an attempt at the universal explanation of the nature of things, said by:**
A. Brightman
B. Henderson
C. Raymond
D. Rousseau

122. **Philosophy is unceasing effort to discern the general truth that lies behind the particular facts, discern also the reality that lies behind appearances, is the opinion of:**
A. Brightman
B. Henderson
C. Raymond
D. Rousseau

123. **The oldest philosophy is:**
A. Idealism
B. Realism
C. Naturalism
D. Theism

124. **Overall development of child is the aim of curriculum belongs to:**
A. Idealistic
B. Naturalistic
C. Realistic
D. Theistic

125. **The prime aim of education, self realization is according to:**
A. Idealism
B. Realism
C. Naturalism
D. Theism

126. **The chief proponents of naturalism is:**
A. Brightman
B. Henderson
C. Raymond
D. Rousseau

127. **The three different form of naturalism are the following, *except:***
A. Physical naturalism
B. Biological naturalism
C. Mechanical naturalism
D. Realistic naturalism

128. **The laws of physical nature govern the laws of human life and adherence to natural laws is essential for human existence, is the belief of:**
A. Physical naturalism
B. Biological naturalism
C. Mechanical naturalism
D. Realistic naturalism

---

121 B 122 C 123 A 124 A 125 A 126 D 127 D
128 A

129. Man being a descendent ape possess animal nature and is devoid of any element of spiritualism, is the view of:
A. Physical naturalism
B. Biological naturalism
C. Mechanical naturalism
D. Realistic naturalism

130. Man as a mere machine devoid of spirit and soul and aims at training man as a good machine is a view of:
A. Physical naturalism
B. Biological naturalism
C. Mechanical naturalism
D. Realistic naturalism

131. Pragmatism originated in:
A. Greece
B. Egypt
C. America
D. Canada

132. Modern pragmatism originated in:
A. Greece
B. Egypt
C. America
D. Canada

133. Proponents of modern pragmatism are the following *except:*
A. Charles Chandus Pierce
B. William James
C. John dewey
D. Ross

134. Pragmatic trend in education is known as:
A. Naturalism
B. Existentialism
C. Eclectism
D. Progressivism

135. Observation and experiment as methods of teaching is advocated by:
A. Idealism
B. Realism
C. Naturalism
D. Pragmatism

136. Social discipline is the belief of:
A. Idealist
B. Realist
C. Naturalist
D. Pragmatist

137. The youngest philosophy is the:
A. Pragmatism
B. Eclectism
C. Supernaturalism
D. Humanistic existentialism

---

129 B 130 C 131 A 132 C 133 D 134 D 135 D
136 D 137 D

138. Supernaturalism is otherwise known as:

A. Pragmatism
B. Eclectism
C. Supernaturalism
D. Theistic realism

139. An assistance available by competent counsellor to an individual to help him direct his own life is the:

A. Guidance
B. Counselling
C. Advice
D. Testing

140. A process of enabling the individual to know himself is the:

A. Guidance
B. Counselling
C. Advice
D. Testing

141. Areas were student require assistance are:

A. Education
B. Personal
C. Financial
D. All

142. An approach in which the counsellor uses variety of techniques to suggest appropriate solution to the problem of counsellee is:

A. Directive counselling
B. Non-directive counselling
C. Eclective counselling
D. None of these

143. An approach in which the counselee is guided to use his own inner resources to solve the problem is the:

A. Directive counselling
B. Non-directive counselling
C. Eclective counselling
D. None of these

144. Directive counselling is also known as:

A. Prescriptive counselling
B. Indirect counselling
C. Counsellee centered counselling
D. Permissive counselling

145. Prescriptive counselling is also known as:

A. Directive counselling
B. Indirect counselling
C. Counsellee centered counselling
D. Permissive counselling

---

138 D 139 A 140 B 141 D 142 A 143 B 144 A
145 C

146. Counsellor centered counselling is otherwise known as:
A. Directive counselling
B. Indirect counselling
C. Counsellee centered counselling
D. Permissive counselling

147. Non-directive counselling is also known as:
A. Permissive counselling
B. Directive counselling
C. Prescriptive counselling
D. Counsellor centered counselling

148. Permissive counselling is otherwise known as:
A. Nondirective counselling
B. Direct counselling
C. Counsellor centered counselling
D. Permissive counselling

149. Client centered counselling also known as:
A. Prescriptive counselling
B. Direct counselling
C. Counsellor centered counselling
D. Permissive counselling

150. The combination of both directive, non-directive and other approaches is the:
A. Eclective counselling
B. Direct counselling
C. Counsellor centered counselling
D. Permissive counselling

151. Phases of counselling are all the following, *except:*
A. Assessment
B. Setting goals
C. Intervention
D. Decision making

152. An approach in which a student, who is misbehaving, is told to stop with the reason is the:
A. Assertive discipline
B. Self discipline
C. True discipline
D. Compulsive discipline

146 A 147 A 148 A 149 D 150 A 151 D 152 A

153. **A combination of self control and self direction is the:**
  A. Assertive discipline
  B. Self discipline
  C. Personal discipline
  D. Compulsive discipline

154. **The lowest level of discipline imposed from the top down is the:**
  A. Assertive discipline
  B. Self discipline
  C. Personal discipline
  D. Compulsive discipline

155. **Self discipline is regarded as:**
  A. Assertive discipline
  B. True discipline
  C. Personal discipline
  D. Compulsive discipline

156. **The discipline centered in the personality of the individual who administers it is the:**
  A. Assertive discipline
  B. Self discipline
  C. Personal discipline
  D. Compulsive discipline

157. **The discipline centered in the group is the:**
  A. Assertive discipline
  B. Self discipline
  C. Social discipline
  D. Compulsive discipline

158. **The curriculum planned by groups outside of an educational institution is the:**
  A. Societal
  B. Institutional
  C. Instructional
  D. Environmental

---

153 B 154 D 155 B 156 C 157 C 158 A

159. The curriculum planned by a faculty for a clearly identified group of students is the:
A. Societal
B. Institutional
C. Instructional
D. Environmental

160. The curriculum consists of the content planned day by day for a particular group of students is the:
A. Societal
B. Institutional
C. Instructional
D. Environmental

161. An essential part of teaching and learning is the:
A. Evaluation
B. Curriculum
C. Objective
D. Philosophy

162. A one, i.e. the process of ascertaining or judging the value of something by careful appraisal is the:
A. Evaluation
B. Curriculum
C. Objective
D. Philosophy

163. Relative and flexible standards are used in:
A. Evaluation
B. Curriculum
C. Objective
D. Philosophy

164. Fixed standards are used in:
A. Evaluation
B. Measurement
C. Objective
D. Philosophy

165. A complete evaluation programme includes are the following, *except:*
A. Educational objective
B. Teaching learning procedures
C. Student progress
D. Teachers progress

166. Formal evaluation is all the following, *except:*
A. Test
B. Rating scale
C. Check list
D. Observation

167. Informal evaluation is all the following, *except:*
A. Observation of students
B. Teachers whole estimate
C. Students reaction to learning
D. Rating scale

---

159 B 160 C 161 A 162 A 163 A 164 B 165 D
166 D 167 D

168. **The major criteria used in selecting and or developing test are all the following, *except:***
   A. Validity B. Reliability
   C. Practicality D. Specificity

169. **The degree of the test to which it measures what it is intended to measure is:**
   A. Validity B. Reliability
   C. Practicality D. Specificity

170. **A test that measures what it is supposed to measure and also measure it accurately is the:**
   A. Validity B. Reliability
   C. Practicality D. Specificity

171. **A one that must be determined by application and by statistical computation is the:**
   A. Validity B. Reliability
   C. Practicality D. Specificity

172. **The criteria refers to the development of evaluative devices capable of being administer is the:**
   A. Validity B. Reliability
   C. Practicality D. Specificity

173. **Test and scales that have met the criteria of testing are known as:**
   A. Standardised test B. Objective test
   C. Subjective test D. Attitude test

174. **A test intended to discover the possibilities of a student's success in some specified one is the:**
   A. Standardised test B. Objective test
   C. Prognostic test D. Attitude test

175. **A test, i.e. designed to indicate the accomplishment of the students in particular subjects is the:**
   A. Standardised test
   B. Achievement test
   C. Prognostic test
   D. Attitude test

---

168 D 169 A 170 B 171 B 172 C 173 A 174 C
175 B

176. A standardized method of recording interpretation of behaviour is the:

A. Test
B. Rating scale
C. Check list
D. Observation

177. The hospital situation with its many and varied activities provide:

A. Direct experience
B. Indirect experience
C. Vicarious experience
D. Symbolic experience

178. Experience through the medium of audio visual materials is the:

A. Direct experience
B. Indirect experience
C. Vicarious experience
D. Symbolic experience

179. Experience through the use of symbols is the:

A. Direct experience
B. Indirect experience
C. Vicarious experience
D. Symbolic experience

180. A thermometer is an example for:

A. Specimen
B. Model
C. Object
D. Mockup

181. A section of a long bone is an example for:

A. Specimen
B. Model
C. Object
D. Mockup

182. Manikin is an example for:

A. Specimen
B. Model
C. Object
D. Mockup

183. Using an artificial kidney to demonstrate dialysis is an example for:

A. Specimen
B. Model
C. Object
D. Mockup

---

176 B 177 A 178 C 179 D 180 C 181 A 182 B
183 D

184. A mold made of plastic material to stimulate some life object is a:
A. Specimen
B. Moulage
C. Object
D. Mockup

185. The following are the fundamental forms of graphic representation, *except:*
A. Graphs
B. Charts
C. Maps
D. Realia

186. Visualization of non-numerical relationship and processes is the:
A. Graphs
B. Charts
C. Maps
D. Realia

187. Graphic representation of the earth's surface are portion of it are termed as:
A. Graphs
B. Charts
C. Maps
D. Realia

188. Visual description that explain rather than represent is the:
A. Diagram
B. Charts
C. Maps
D. Realia

189. A vehicle for a variety of visual materials is the:
A. Poster
B. Chalk board
C. Bulletin board
D. Flannel board

190. A runway for attaining the goals of education is the:
A. Curriculum
B. Syllabus
C. Objective
D. Philosophy

191. The Latin word currere means:
A. Run
B. Lead
C. Go
D. Hold

192. As per the definition given by Cunningham for curriculum, the artist refers to:
A. Teacher
B. Material
C. Ideals
D. Studio

---

184 B 185 D 186 B 187 C 188 A 189 B 190 A
191 A 192 A

193. As per the definition given by Cunningham for curriculum, the material refers to:

A. Teacher
B. Students
C. Ideals
D. Studio

194. As per the definition given by Cunningham for curriculum, the ideals refers to:

A. Teacher
B. Material
C. Objective
D. Studio

195. As per the definition given by Cunningham for curriculum, the studio refers to:

A. Teacher
B. Material
C. Ideals
D. Educational institution

196. The oldest method of teaching is the:

A. Lecture
B. Discussion
C. Conference
D. Seminar

197. Psychomotor skills in teaching is used in:

A. Lecture
B. Demonstration
C. Conference
D. Seminar

198. Seminar conducted in the classroom is called:

A. Mini seminar
B. Main seminar
C. National seminar
D. International seminar

199. Seminar organized at the institutional level is the:

A. Mini seminar
B. Main seminar
C. National seminar
D. International seminar

200. A teacher's education technique is the:

A. Micro teaching
B. Macro teaching
C. Classroom teaching
D. Clinical teaching

201. A plan proposed by a teacher to take class is:

A. Unit plan
B. Course plan
C. Lesson plan
D. Master plan

202. The type of evaluation done after the completion of curriculum is:

A. Formative evaluation
B. Summative evaluation
C. Scientific evaluation
D. Program evaluation

---

193 B 194 C 195 D 196 A 197 B 198 A 199 B
200 A 201 C 202 B

203. An educational communication media that provide an opportunity for situational learning is:
A. Field trip
B. Specimen
C. Module
D. Chart

204. The principles to be followed in counseling includes all, except:
A. Acceptance
B. Guidance
C. Reassurance
D. Avoidance

205. An institution which is systematically organized and set up:
A. Formal
B. Informal
C. Social
D. Civil

206. The following are the processes of human communication, except:
A. Source
B. Message
C. Channel
D. Sound

207. Panel discussion consists of ________ members:
A. 4–8
B. 9–11
C. 12–15
D. 16–18

208. Clarification of facts is possible in:
A. Lecture
B. Seminar
C. Work shop
D. Panel discussion

209. The term kindergarten represents:
A. Primary
B. Secondary
C. Higher secondary
D. Lower and upper

210. The receiver of message is also known:
A. Decoder
B. Encoder
C. Recorder
D. Feed backer

211. The written report of verbal interaction with patients is:
A. Feed back
B. Process recording
C. Anecdotal record
D. Report

212. The process of growth and development of learner is:
A. Teaching
B. Learning
C. Discussing
D. Thinking

203 A 204 D 205 A 206 D 207 A 208 A
209 D 210 A 211 B 212 D

213. One day per week completely for theory hours in a teaching system is:
A. Study day
B. Partial block
C. Complete block
D. Split teaching

214. A planned educational experience provided to an employee at the job setting is:
A. Inservice education
B. Orientation
C. Workshop
D. Counseling

215. The one that helps to improve the knowledge, skill and attitude of employees is:
A. Workshop
B. Adult education
C. Conference
D. Staff development program

216. Minimum age of entry into BSc (N) course is:
A. 17 years
B. 19 years
C. 20 years
D. Any age

217. Laying of minimum standard of education in nursing is the responsibility of:
A. University
B. Government
C. State Council
D. Indian Nursing Council

218. Reporting a specific event that occurred in the clinical area is:
A. Legal report
B. Incident report
C. Transfer report
D. Nurses report

219. The following are the legal safeguards in nursing practice, except:
A. Licensure
B. Standing order
C. Oral report
D. Informed consent

220. Written record of duties and responsibilities is:
A. Job description
B. Job analysis
C. Job specification
D. Job evaluation

221. A single sheet of paper folded to make a full page of printed material is called:
A. Pamphlet
B. Handout
C. Leaflet
D. Booklet

---

213 A 214 A 215 D 216 A 217 D 218 B 219 C
220 A 221 A

222. An electronic device, in which sound and light energy are transmitted from one place to another is:
A. Television
B. Radio
C. Computer
D. Telescope

223. A test that measures the attainments on accomplishments of learner after a period of learning is:
A. Teacher made test
B. Achievement test
C. Attitude test
D. Aptitude test

224. The psychomotor domain denotes:
A Knowledge
B. Attitude
C. Skills
D. Interest

225. The cognitive domain denotes:
A. Knowledge
B. Attitude
C. Skills
D. Interest

226. The affective domain denotes:
A. Knowledge
B. Attitude
C. Skills
D. Interest

227. A person who seeks help or needs assistance is:
A. Counselor
B. Counselee
C. Advisor
D. Guides

228. The table that shows the schedule for group activity is:
A. Flow chart
B. Tabulation chart
C. Time table
D. Flip chart

229. A verbal snap shot of an incident is called:
A. Anecdotal
B. Checklist
C. Rating scale
D. Incident

230. A basic tool for counseling is:
A. Exam
B. Records
C. Interview
D. Talking

231. The basis of sensitivity training, sociodrama, role playing and psychodrama is:
A. Simulation
B. Seminar
C. Lecture
D. Microteaching

222 A 223 B 224 C 225 A 226 B 227 B
228 C 229 A 230 D 231 A

232. The group of individuals who work together towards the solution of problems in a given subject matter field during a specific period of time is called:

A. Penal B. Seminar
C. Symposium D. Workshop

233. The scaled down sample of teaching is called:

A. Simulation B. Demonstration
C. Lecture D. Microteaching

234. The word cognition means:

A. Knowing B. Feeling
C. Doing D. Listening

235. Love of wisdom denotes:

A. Philosophy B. Psychology
C. Physiology D. Sociology

236. Pragmatism means:

A. Knowledge B. Facts
C. Practice D. Application

237. Education is _______ Philosophy:

A. Dynamic B. Social
C. Stable D. Current

238. An example of non-projected visual aid is:

A. Flashcards B. Slides
C. Filmstrip D. Television

239. Essay type of question is the assessment of:

A. Skill B. Altitude
C. Knowledge D. Emotion

240. The one that gives the student's details in the college is:

A. Cumulative record
B. Health record
C. Assessment register
D. Admission register

---

232 D 233 D 234 A 235 A 236 C 237 A 238 A
239 C 240 A

241. **The four components of communication are:**
   A. Ideas, facts, feelings and information
   B. Source, message, channel and receiver
   C. Oral, sign, action and object
   D. Channel, action, message and ideas

242. **An educational technique that involves acting art of a problem is:**
   A. Project method B. Role play
   C. Assignment D. Conference

243. **The method teaches by exhibition and exploration is:**
   A. Discussion B. Clinical teaching
   C. Case study D. Demonstration

244. **An exact written report of the conversation between nurse and the patient is:**
   A. Process recording B. Nurse's report
   C. Nurse's record D. Progress record

245. **The one that projects the transparencies image on the screen is:**
   A. Slide projector B. Over head projector
   C. Television D. Epidiascope

246. **The size of the flash card is:**
   A. 23″ x 30″ B. 22″ x 28″
   C. 28″ x 30″ D. 20″ x 25″

247. **Learning directly through personal experience in nature is:**
   A. Naturalism B. Idealism
   C. Realism D. Pragmatism

248. **The act of giving advice is:**
   A. Guidance B. Counseling
   C. Discussion D. Interview

249. **The principle to be followed in counseling is:**
   A. Observation B. Questioning
   C. Restatement D. Acceptance

250. **Puppet show promotes:**
   A. Creative ability B. Self-awareness
   C. Self-interest D. Skills

---

241 B 242 B 243 D 244 A 245 B 246 D 247 A
248 A 249 A 250 A

251. The techniques of therapeutic communication is:
A. Awareness
B. Acceptance
C. Humor
D. Trust

252. Natural learning method is:
A. Field trip
B. Role play
C. Sociodrama
D. Simulation

253. The method of teaching useful for self-faced learning is:
A. Lecture
B. Demonstration
C. Program instruction
D. Computer-assisted instruction.

254. The component of therapeutic relationship is:
A. Acceptance
B. Warmth
C. Accountability
D. Confidentiality

255. The element that hinders counseling process is:
A. Confidentiality
B. Trust
C. Passing moral judgments
D. Running comments

256. Barrier to effective communication is:
A. Educational difference
B. Language
C. Culture
D. Ability

257. In teaching and learning process the activities includes:
A. Planning, organizing, leading and controlling
B. Intelligence, motivation, attitude and learning
C. Lecturing, demonstrating, experimenting and knowing
D. None of these

258. Use of chalk boards, maps, charts, etc. is known as:
A. Exhibits
B. Visual aid
C. Audio aid
D. Still pictures

259. The test that assess the knowledge of students accurately is:
A. Objective test
B. Subjective test
C. Skill test
D. Practical test

---

251 D 252 A 253 D 254 D 255 D 256 B 257 A
258 B 259 A

260. By education 'I mean all round drawing out of the best' is said by:

A. Mahatma Gandhi
B. Socrates
C. Radha Krishnan
D. Tagore

261. The one not an element of a learning process is:

A. Perception
B. Stimuli
C. Integration
D. Philosophy

262. The method of teaching, which is to test, analyze and prepare the various chemicals is:

A. Demonstration
B. Discussion
C. Laboratory
D. Conference

263. Intelligence test is done to assess:

A. Trait
B. Personality
C. Learning capacity
D. Interest

264. An objective, i.e. is stated in relation to learners desired outcome is:

A. Behavior centered
B. Learner centered
C. Subject centered
D. Teacher centered

265. The philosophy of education rests upon:

A. Philosophy of life
B. Theistic realism
C. Leorealism
D. Idealism

266. As per Indian nursing council (INC), the total bed occupancy of a hospital to run college of nursing should be:

A. 50%
B. 60%
C. 70%
D. 75%

267. Mental activity by means of which knowledge, skill, attitude appreciation and ideas are acquired in:

A. Education
B. Philosophy
C. Learning
D. Teaching

268. The following are the role function of a nursing teaching except:

A. Instructional role
B. Faculty role
C. Individual role
D. Managerial role

---

260 A 261 D 262 C 263 C 264 A 265 A 266 D
267 C 268 D

269. **The philosophy that applies the theories of sciences in solving problem is:**
   A. Idealism
   B. Naturalism
   C. Pragmatism
   D. Realism

270. **Project method of learning is an important component of:**
   A. Idealism
   B. Naturalism
   C. Pragmatism
   D. Realism

271. **The three levels of curriculum planning are the following, except:**
   A. Social
   B. Institutional
   C. Instructional
   D. Individual

272. **The visual presentation of the action and activities related to the facts and principles of the delivered lesson is:**
   A. Problem solving
   B. Role play
   C. Demonstration
   D. Field visit

273. **Collection of real thing for teaching purpose refers to:**
   A. Model
   B. Specimen
   C. Objects
   D. Mock

274. **Naturalist believe in:**
   A. God
   B. Material
   C. Nature
   D. Practice

275. **The methods used to assess the knowledge are the following, except:**
   A. Subjective test
   B. Objective test
   C. Problem solving
   D. Anecdotal

276. **Programmed instruction is:**
   A. Individualized technique
   B. Group technique
   C. Student technique
   D. Subject technique

277. **Counseling process has:**
   A. 3 phases
   B. 4 phases
   C. 5 phases
   D. 6 phases

---

269 D 270 C 271 D 272 C 273 B 274 C 275 D
276 A 277 C

278. **The time to be taken in nursing rounds for each patient is:**
A. 4 minutes
B. 10 minutes
C. 15 minutes
D. 20 minutes

279. **Factors to be considered in planning a unit are the following, except:**
A. Objectives
B. Content
C. Learning activities
D. Teacher

280. **A revision on repetition, of the knowledge learnt in the lesson is known as:**
A. Application
B. Generalization
C. Recapitulation
D. Presentation

281. **The first activity in a planning unit is:**
A. Selection of content
B. Selection of methods of evaluation
C. Selection of reference
D. Selection of statements of objectives

282. **The selection of learning experiences is dependent on:**
A. Type of program
B. Climate
C. Reference
D. Teacher

283. **Data necessary for formulation of educational objective is:**
A. Health needs of society
B. Economic status of the society
C. Religious activities of the society
D. Cultural activities of the society.

284. **Curriculum evaluation is done on the following, except:**
A. Teaching learning process
B. Student outcomes
C. Use of audio visual (AV) aids
D. Organization

285. **The teacher-student ratio prescribed by INC is:**
A. 1:10
B. 1:5
C. 1:15
D. 1:20

278 A 279 D 280 C 281 D 282 A 283 A 284 D
285 A

286. The Student-patient ratio prescribed by INC is:

A. 1:3
B. 1:1
C. 1:2
D. 1:5

287. The plan that shows classroom teaching and clinical experience is:

A. Course plan
B. Master plan
C. Unit plan
D. Clinic rotation plan

288. To setup a new school of nursing, no-objection certificate to be obtained from:

A. State Government
B. INC
C. University
D. State Council

289. The role of university in nursing collegiate program in all the following, except:

A. Examination
B. Registration
C. Issue of degree
D. Disciplinary action

290. In Tamil Nadu, the examination for Diploma in Nursing program is conducted by:

A. University
B. State Council
C. Board
D. None of these

291. Advisory Committee is set up at the level of:

A. Controlling authority
B. Faculty authority
C. Administrative authority
D. All of these

292. Advise on monitoring and evaluation of nursing program is the function of:

A. Advisory Committee
B. Curriculum Committee
C. Co-curricular Committee
D. Selection Committee

293. Recruitment and selection of students is done by:

A. Curriculum Committee
B. Discipline Committee
C. Selection Committee
D. Welfare Committee

---

286 A 287 B 288 A 289 D 290 C 291 A 292 A
293 C

294. **The following are the components of curriculum, except:**
A. Philosophy
B. Objectives
C. Evaluation
D. Recruitment

295. **In determining the objectives, the following factors should be considered, except:**
A. Philosophy
B. Role of nurse
C. Infrastructure resources
D. Remuneration for staff

296. **The components of the total program should be evaluated are:**
A. Philosophy
B. Finance
C. Curriculum
D. All of these

297. **In students performance evaluation, the principle of which needs to be kept in mind is:**
A. Individual difference
B. Teaching and learning
C. Curriculum
D. Administration

298. **Assignment is the method of assessing:**
A. Attitude
B. Skill
C. Both
D. None of these

299. **The academic qualification needed to get admission into diploma nursing program is:**
A. +2 with science
B. +2 with any subject
C. +2 with vocation group
D. 10th pass

300. **Getting an official authorization to run a nursing educational institution is:**
A. Affiliation
B. Accreditation
C. Organization
D. Appreciation

---

294 D 295 D 296 D 297 A 298 A 299 B 300 B